Parkinson's Fall & Freezing Logbook

90 Days Logbook Tracking Falls, Freezing Episodes & Triggers | A Safety & Prevention Journal for Parkinson's Caregivers

Daniel Harper

Helping caregivers stay organized, informed, and supported

AF720583

Medical Disclaimer

This journal is intended for personal organization and caregiving support. It is not a substitute for professional medical advice, diagnosis, or treatment

Message to Caregivers

To the Caregiver

If you are using this logbook, it likely means you are caring for someone living with Parkinson's. That role requires patience, strength, and compassion every single day.

This book was created to make that journey a little easier by helping you track important information, recognize health patterns, and stay organized during medical visits.

More importantly, it is a reminder that you do not have to carry every detail alone.

Your care matters.
Your effort matters.
And the support you provide makes a real difference.

Table of Contents

Introduction 5
How To Use This Logbook 7
Section 1 - Quick Reference Page 10
Red Flag Alerts 13
Section 2 - Fall Incident Tracker 16
Section 3 - Freezing Episode Tracker 47
Section 4 - Daily Safety Check & Risk Rating 72
Section 5 - Weekly Safety Summary & Pattern Insights 118
Section 10 - Doctor Visits & Medical Notes 143
Final 90-Day Safety Summary & Care Insights 157
Closing Message for Caregivers 161
A Small Request From the Author 162

Introduction

Safety in Parkinson's care begins with awareness.

Falls and freezing episodes are among the most challenging and potentially dangerous, symptoms of Parkinson's disease. They can occur without warning, disrupt daily life, and lead to serious injuries, hospitalizations, and loss of confidence for both patients and caregivers.

For many caregivers, the uncertainty is the hardest part.

- *Why did this fall happen?*
- *What caused the freezing episode?*
- *How can it be prevented next time?*

Without clear tracking, these questions often go unanswered.

Why This Logbook Matters

The truth is, most falls and freezing episodes are **not random**. They are often linked to patterns such as:

- Specific times of day
- Medication "wearing off" periods
- Environmental triggers (doorways, clutter, poor lighting)
- Fatigue or stress

When these patterns are identified, risks can be reduced.

This logbook is designed to help you move from uncertainty to clarity by giving you a simple, structured way to record, observe, and understand what is happening.

What This Book Helps You Do

With consistent use, this logbook will help you:

- Track falls and freezing episodes in detail
- Identify common triggers and high-risk situations
- Monitor changes over time
- Improve communication with healthcare provider
- Take proactive steps to enhance safety

A Tool for Prevention, Not Just Recording

This is more than a logbook, it is a **safety and prevention tool**.

Every entry you make helps build a clearer picture of:

- When risks are highest
- What situations should be avoided or modified
- What strategies are working

Over time, this information becomes incredibly valuable in preventing future incidents.

A Note to Caregivers

Caring for someone with Parkinson's requires patience, vigilance, and strength. Managing fall risk and freezing episodes can feel overwhelming, but you are not alone in this journey.

Your observations matter.
Your consistency matters.
Your care makes a difference every single day.

Small observations can prevent serious events.
And prevention is one of the most powerful forms of care.

How To Use This Logbook

A Simple System to Track, Understand & Prevent Falls and Freezing Episodes

This logbook is designed to help you **identify patterns, reduce risks, and improve safety** for individuals living with Parkinson's disease.

You do not need to fill out every section perfectly.
Consistency matters more than perfection.

STEP 1 , START WITH THE QUICK REFERENCE PAGE

Begin by completing the **Quick Reference Page** at the front of the book.

This includes:

- Patient details
- Emergency contacts
- Mobility status
- Known triggers

This page provides a **snapshot of current condition and risks**.

STEP 2 , RECORD EVERY FALL

Each time a fall occurs, complete a **Fall Incident Report**.

Be sure to note:

- Date and time
- Location and activity
- Possible cause or trigger
- Type of fall and any injuries

Even small details can help identify patterns and prevent future incidents.

STEP 3 , TRACK FREEZING EPISODES

Freezing can happen suddenly and often leads to falls.

Record each episode with:

- Time and duration
- Activity during the episode
- Trigger (if known)
- Severity and assistance needed

Over time, you may notice **repeat triggers** such as turning, doorways, or fatigue.

STEP 4 , USE THE DAILY SAFETY CHECK (OPTIONAL)

At the end of each day, complete the **Daily Safety Check**.

This helps you quickly record:

- Whether any falls or freezing occurred
- Overall safety level for the day
- Risk factors like fatigue or medication timing

This step takes less than a minute but adds valuable daily insight.

STEP 5 , COMPLETE WEEKLY SUMMARY

At the end of each week, fill in the **Weekly Safety Summary**.

Focus on:

- Total falls and freezing episodes
- Most common triggers
- High-risk times of day
- Overall safety trend

This is where patterns become clear.

STEP 6 , REVIEW YOUR FINAL SUMMARY

At the end of the logbook, complete the **Final 90-Day Summary**.

This helps you:

- See long-term patterns
- Identify improvements or concerns
- Prepare for doctor visits

Bring this summary to appointments for **better, more informed care decisions**.

HELPFUL TIPS FOR BEST RESULTS

✓ Record events as soon as possible while details are fresh
✓ Be honest and consistent, there is no "perfect" entry
✓ Look for patterns, not isolated incidents
✓ Share your notes with healthcare providers
✓ Use insights to make small safety improvements at home

A NOTE TO CAREGIVERS

Managing fall risk and freezing episodes can feel unpredictable, but tracking brings clarity.

Every entry you make helps:

- Improve safety
- Reduce risk
- Build confidence in caregiving

You are doing important, meaningful work.
And this logbook is here to support you every step of the way.

Section 1 - Quick Reference Page

(Fall & Freezing Safety Overview)

Patient Information

- Full Name: ____
- Date of Birth: _____________________________________
- Diagnosis Date: ___________________________________
- Primary Care Physician: ____________________________
- Neurologist / Specialist: ___________________________

Emergency Contacts

- Name: ________________________ Phone: _____________
- Name: ________________________ Phone: _____________
- Preferred Hospital: _________________________________

Mobility & Fall Risk Status

- Walks independently: ☐ Yes ☐ No
- Requires assistance: ☐ Sometimes ☐ Always
- Uses mobility aid: ☐ Cane ☐ Walker ☐ Wheelchair ☐ None

Current Fall Risk Level

☐ Low Risk ☐ Moderate Risk ☐ High Risk

Freezing Episodes Overview

- Frequency: ☐ None ☐ Rare ☐ Occasional ☐ Frequent

- Typical situations:
  ☐ Turning ☐ Starting movement ☐ Doorways
  ☐ Crowded spaces ☐ Stress or anxiety ☐ Fatigue

Other: ____

Recent Fall History

- Falls in last 30 days: ______
- Near-falls: ______

Common causes or patterns:

Environmental Risk Factors

☐ Poor lighting
☐ Cluttered walkways
☐ Slippery floors
☐ Uneven surfaces
☐ Stairs without support

Other: ____

Current Medications

Medication Name	Dosage	Time(s)	Purpose	Notes

Medication Notes (Fall/Freezing Related)

- Medication taken regularly: ☐ Yes ☐ No
- Wearing-off periods noticed: ☐ Yes ☐ No

Time of highest risk (if known):

Key Triggers to Watch

☐ Fatigue
☐ Sudden movement
☐ Distractions
☐ Anxiety or stress
☐ Medication delay

Other: ____

Important Safety Notes

Doctor Instructions / Recommendations

QUICK REMINDER

High-risk times and triggers can change.
Review and update this page regularly to keep care safe and effective.

Red Flag Alerts

When to Seek Immediate Help or Contact Your Doctor

Falls and freezing episodes can sometimes signal **serious underlying risks**. Recognizing warning signs early can help prevent injury and ensure timely medical care.

CALL EMERGENCY SERVICES IMMEDIATELY

Seek urgent medical attention if the patient experiences:

- A fall with **head injury** or loss of consciousness
- Inability to get up after a fall
- Severe pain after a fall (possible fracture)
- Sudden inability to move, stand, or speak
- Signs of stroke (face drooping, arm weakness, slurred speech)
- Difficulty breathing or chest pain
- Seizures or uncontrollable shaking beyond normal tremors

CONTACT YOUR DOCTOR PROMPTLY

Movement & Safety Concerns

- Frequent or repeated falls within a short period
- Sudden increase in freezing episodes
- Freezing episodes lasting longer than usual
- Noticeable decline in balance or walking ability

Freezing Episode Changes

- Freezing occurring in new situations
- Episodes triggered more easily than before

- Increased difficulty restarting movement

Medication-Related Issues

- Medication "wearing off" much earlier than expected
- Medication not improving symptoms
- Sudden increase in OFF periods
- New or severe involuntary movements (dyskinesia)
- Missed doses leading to significant symptom worsening

Cognitive & Behavioural Changes

- Sudden confusion or disorientation
- Hallucinations or unusual behavior
- Increased anxiety, agitation, or fear of walking

General Health Concerns

- Persistent fatigue or weakness
- Dizziness or fainting
- Difficulty swallowing (risk of choking)
- Signs of infection (fever, cough, urinary issues)

CAREGIVER ACTION NOTES

If a red flag occurs, record details clearly:

- Date & time: ______________________________
- What happened: ____________________________
- Possible trigger: __________________________
- Medication taken prior: ____________________
- Duration of symptoms: _____________________
- Action taken: _____________________________

A NOTE TO CAREGIVERS

You know the person you care for better than anyone.
If something feels unusual or concerning—**trust your instincts**.

It is always better to **seek help early** than to wait.

REMINDER

Tracking patterns helps prevent risks—but **acting on warning signs protects lives**.

Section 2 - Fall Incident Tracker

(Detailed Fall Recording for Safety & Prevention)

Purpose of This Section

Every fall provides important information.
Recording the details helps you **identify patterns, reduce risk, and prevent future incidents**.

Record every episode of fall when it happens

Complete this page immediately after any fall or near-fall.

FALL INCIDENT REPORT

Date: ____________________ **Time:** ____________________

LOCATION

Where did the fall occur?

☐ Bedroom ☐ Bathroom ☐ Living room ☐ Kitchen
☐ Outdoors ☐ Stairs Other: ________________________________

ACTIVITY AT THE TIME

What was the person doing?

☐ Walking ☐ Turning ☐ Standing up ☐ Sitting down
☐ Reaching for something ☐ Using stairs Other: __________

TYPE OF FALL

☐ Forward ☐ Backward ☐ Sideways ☐ Slipped
☐ Lost balance ☐ Unknown

WAS FREEZING INVOLVED?

☐ Yes ☐ No ☐ Unsure

If yes, describe:

POSSIBLE CAUSE / TRIGGER

☐ Loss of balance ☐ Freezing episode ☐ Fatigue

☐ Slippery surface ☐ Poor lighting ☐ Clutter / obstacle

☐ Medication wearing off Other: ____

INJURY DETAILS

☐ No injury ☐ Minor (bruises, soreness) ☐ Moderate (pain, swelling)
☐ Severe (possible fracture, head injury) **Body area affected:** _________

ASSISTANCE REQUIRED

☐ None ☐ Help from caregiver
☐ Medical attention needed Details: ___________________________________

MEDICATION STATUS

- Medication taken on time? ☐ Yes ☐ No
- Time since last dose: ______________ Wearing-off noticed? ☐ Yes ☐ No

---

ENVIRONMENTAL FACTORS

☐ Poor lighting ☐ Wet/slippery floor ☐ Uneven surface ☐ Cluttered area

Other: ____

NOTES & OBSERVATIONS

What stood out about this incident?

INCIDENT SEVERITY RATING

☐ Low Risk ☐ Moderate Risk ☐ High Risk

PREVENTIVE ACTION (IMPORTANT)

What can be done to reduce future risk?

☐ Improve lighting
☐ Remove obstacles
☐ Adjust medication timing
☐ Increase supervision
☐ Use mobility aid

Other: ____

QUICK REMINDER

Every recorded fall helps build a clearer picture.
Patterns identified today can **prevent serious injuries tomorrow**.

FALL INCIDENT REPORT

Date: ____________________ **Time:** ____________________

LOCATION

Where did the fall occur?

☐ Bedroom ☐ Bathroom ☐ Living room ☐ Kitchen
☐ Outdoors ☐ Stairs Other: ________________________________

ACTIVITY AT THE TIME

What was the person doing?

☐ Walking ☐ Turning ☐ Standing up ☐ Sitting down
☐ Reaching for something ☐ Using stairs Other: __________

TYPE OF FALL

☐ Forward ☐ Backward ☐ Sideways ☐ Slipped
☐ Lost balance ☐ Unknown

WAS FREEZING INVOLVED?

☐ Yes ☐ No ☐ Unsure

If yes, describe:

POSSIBLE CAUSE / TRIGGER

☐ Loss of balance ☐ Freezing episode ☐ Fatigue

☐ Slippery surface ☐ Poor lighting ☐ Clutter / obstacle

☐ Medication wearing off Other: ______________________________________

INJURY DETAILS

☐ No injury ☐ Minor (bruises, soreness) ☐ Moderate (pain, swelling)
☐ Severe (possible fracture, head injury) **Body area affected:** _________

ASSISTANCE REQUIRED

☐ None ☐ Help from caregiver
☐ Medical attention needed Details: ________________________________

MEDICATION STATUS

- Medication taken on time? ☐ Yes ☐ No
- Time since last dose: _______________ Wearing-off noticed? ☐ Yes ☐ No

---

ENVIRONMENTAL FACTORS

☐ Poor lighting ☐ Wet/slippery floor ☐ Uneven surface ☐ Cluttered area

Other: ____

NOTES & OBSERVATIONS

What stood out about this incident?

INCIDENT SEVERITY RATING

☐ Low Risk ☐ Moderate Risk ☐ High Risk

PREVENTIVE ACTION (IMPORTANT)

What can be done to reduce future risk?

☐ Improve lighting
☐ Remove obstacles
☐ Adjust medication timing
☐ Increase supervision
☐ Use mobility aid

Other: ____

QUICK REMINDER

Every recorded fall helps build a clearer picture.
Patterns identified today can **prevent serious injuries tomorrow**.

FALL INCIDENT REPORT

Date: ____________________ **Time:** ____________________

LOCATION

Where did the fall occur?

☐ Bedroom ☐ Bathroom ☐ Living room ☐ Kitchen
☐ Outdoors ☐ Stairs Other: ________________________________

ACTIVITY AT THE TIME

What was the person doing?

☐ Walking ☐ Turning ☐ Standing up ☐ Sitting down
☐ Reaching for something ☐ Using stairs Other: __________

TYPE OF FALL

☐ Forward ☐ Backward ☐ Sideways ☐ Slipped
☐ Lost balance ☐ Unknown

WAS FREEZING INVOLVED?

☐ Yes ☐ No ☐ Unsure

If yes, describe:

POSSIBLE CAUSE / TRIGGER

☐ Loss of balance ☐ Freezing episode ☐ Fatigue

☐ Slippery surface ☐ Poor lighting ☐ Clutter / obstacle

☐ Medication wearing off Other: ____

INJURY DETAILS

☐ No injury ☐ Minor (bruises, soreness) ☐ Moderate (pain, swelling)
☐ Severe (possible fracture, head injury) **Body area affected:** _________

ASSISTANCE REQUIRED

☐ None ☐ Help from caregiver
☐ Medical attention needed Details: ___________________________________

MEDICATION STATUS

- Medication taken on time? ☐ Yes ☐ No
- Time since last dose: _______________ Wearing-off noticed? ☐ Yes ☐ No

---

ENVIRONMENTAL FACTORS

☐ Poor lighting ☐ Wet/slippery floor ☐ Uneven surface ☐ Cluttered area

Other: ____

NOTES & OBSERVATIONS

What stood out about this incident?

INCIDENT SEVERITY RATING

☐ Low Risk ☐ Moderate Risk ☐ High Risk

PREVENTIVE ACTION (IMPORTANT)

What can be done to reduce future risk?

☐ Improve lighting
☐ Remove obstacles
☐ Adjust medication timing
☐ Increase supervision
☐ Use mobility aid

Other: ____

QUICK REMINDER

Every recorded fall helps build a clearer picture.
Patterns identified today can **prevent serious injuries tomorrow**.

FALL INCIDENT REPORT

Date: ____________________ **Time:** ____________________

LOCATION

Where did the fall occur?

☐ Bedroom ☐ Bathroom ☐ Living room ☐ Kitchen
☐ Outdoors ☐ Stairs Other: ________________________________

ACTIVITY AT THE TIME

What was the person doing?

☐ Walking ☐ Turning ☐ Standing up ☐ Sitting down
☐ Reaching for something ☐ Using stairs Other: __________

TYPE OF FALL

☐ Forward ☐ Backward ☐ Sideways ☐ Slipped
☐ Lost balance ☐ Unknown

WAS FREEZING INVOLVED?

☐ Yes ☐ No ☐ Unsure

If yes, describe:

POSSIBLE CAUSE / TRIGGER

☐ Loss of balance ☐ Freezing episode ☐ Fatigue

☐ Slippery surface ☐ Poor lighting ☐ Clutter / obstacle

☐ Medication wearing off Other: ________________________________

INJURY DETAILS

☐ No injury ☐ Minor (bruises, soreness) ☐ Moderate (pain, swelling)
☐ Severe (possible fracture, head injury) **Body area affected:** _________

ASSISTANCE REQUIRED

☐ None ☐ Help from caregiver
☐ Medical attention needed Details: ________________________________

MEDICATION STATUS

- Medication taken on time? ☐ Yes ☐ No
- Time since last dose: _______________ Wearing-off noticed? ☐ Yes ☐ No

---

ENVIRONMENTAL FACTORS

☐ Poor lighting ☐ Wet/slippery floor ☐ Uneven surface ☐ Cluttered area

Other: ____

NOTES & OBSERVATIONS

What stood out about this incident?

INCIDENT SEVERITY RATING

☐ Low Risk ☐ Moderate Risk ☐ High Risk

PREVENTIVE ACTION (IMPORTANT)

What can be done to reduce future risk?

☐ Improve lighting
☐ Remove obstacles
☐ Adjust medication timing
☐ Increase supervision
☐ Use mobility aid

Other: ____

QUICK REMINDER

Every recorded fall helps build a clearer picture.
Patterns identified today can **prevent serious injuries tomorrow**.

FALL INCIDENT REPORT

Date: ____________________ **Time:** ____________________

LOCATION

Where did the fall occur?

☐ Bedroom ☐ Bathroom ☐ Living room ☐ Kitchen
☐ Outdoors ☐ Stairs Other: ________________________________

ACTIVITY AT THE TIME

What was the person doing?

☐ Walking ☐ Turning ☐ Standing up ☐ Sitting down
☐ Reaching for something ☐ Using stairs Other: __________

TYPE OF FALL

☐ Forward ☐ Backward ☐ Sideways ☐ Slipped
☐ Lost balance ☐ Unknown

WAS FREEZING INVOLVED?

☐ Yes ☐ No ☐ Unsure

If yes, describe:

POSSIBLE CAUSE / TRIGGER

☐ Loss of balance ☐ Freezing episode ☐ Fatigue

☐ Slippery surface ☐ Poor lighting ☐ Clutter / obstacle

☐ Medication wearing off Other: ____

INJURY DETAILS

☐ No injury ☐ Minor (bruises, soreness) ☐ Moderate (pain, swelling)
☐ Severe (possible fracture, head injury) **Body area affected:** _________

ASSISTANCE REQUIRED

☐ None ☐ Help from caregiver
☐ Medical attention needed Details: ___________________________________

MEDICATION STATUS

- Medication taken on time? ☐ Yes ☐ No
- Time since last dose: _______________ Wearing-off noticed? ☐ Yes ☐ No

---

ENVIRONMENTAL FACTORS

☐ Poor lighting ☐ Wet/slippery floor ☐ Uneven surface ☐ Cluttered area

Other: ____

NOTES & OBSERVATIONS

What stood out about this incident?

INCIDENT SEVERITY RATING

☐ Low Risk ☐ Moderate Risk ☐ High Risk

PREVENTIVE ACTION (IMPORTANT)

What can be done to reduce future risk?

☐ Improve lighting
☐ Remove obstacles
☐ Adjust medication timing
☐ Increase supervision
☐ Use mobility aid

Other: ____

QUICK REMINDER

Every recorded fall helps build a clearer picture.
Patterns identified today can **prevent serious injuries tomorrow**.

FALL INCIDENT REPORT

Date: ____________________ **Time:** ____________________

LOCATION

Where did the fall occur?

☐ Bedroom ☐ Bathroom ☐ Living room ☐ Kitchen
☐ Outdoors ☐ Stairs Other: ________________________________

ACTIVITY AT THE TIME

What was the person doing?

☐ Walking ☐ Turning ☐ Standing up ☐ Sitting down
☐ Reaching for something ☐ Using stairs Other: __________

TYPE OF FALL

☐ Forward ☐ Backward ☐ Sideways ☐ Slipped
☐ Lost balance ☐ Unknown

WAS FREEZING INVOLVED?

☐ Yes ☐ No ☐ Unsure

If yes, describe:

POSSIBLE CAUSE / TRIGGER

☐ Loss of balance ☐ Freezing episode ☐ Fatigue

☐ Slippery surface ☐ Poor lighting ☐ Clutter / obstacle

☐ Medication wearing off Other: ____

INJURY DETAILS

☐ No injury ☐ Minor (bruises, soreness) ☐ Moderate (pain, swelling)
☐ Severe (possible fracture, head injury) **Body area affected:** _________

ASSISTANCE REQUIRED

☐ None ☐ Help from caregiver
☐ Medical attention needed Details: ___________________________________

MEDICATION STATUS

- Medication taken on time? ☐ Yes ☐ No
- Time since last dose: _______________ Wearing-off noticed? ☐ Yes ☐ No

---

ENVIRONMENTAL FACTORS

☐ Poor lighting ☐ Wet/slippery floor ☐ Uneven surface ☐ Cluttered area

Other: ____

NOTES & OBSERVATIONS

What stood out about this incident?

INCIDENT SEVERITY RATING

☐ Low Risk ☐ Moderate Risk ☐ High Risk

PREVENTIVE ACTION (IMPORTANT)

What can be done to reduce future risk?

☐ Improve lighting
☐ Remove obstacles
☐ Adjust medication timing
☐ Increase supervision
☐ Use mobility aid

Other: ____

QUICK REMINDER

Every recorded fall helps build a clearer picture.
Patterns identified today can **prevent serious injuries tomorrow**.

FALL INCIDENT REPORT

Date: ____________________ **Time:** ____________________

LOCATION

Where did the fall occur?

☐ Bedroom ☐ Bathroom ☐ Living room ☐ Kitchen
☐ Outdoors ☐ Stairs Other: ________________________________

ACTIVITY AT THE TIME

What was the person doing?

☐ Walking ☐ Turning ☐ Standing up ☐ Sitting down
☐ Reaching for something ☐ Using stairs Other: __________

TYPE OF FALL

☐ Forward ☐ Backward ☐ Sideways ☐ Slipped
☐ Lost balance ☐ Unknown

WAS FREEZING INVOLVED?

☐ Yes ☐ No ☐ Unsure

If yes, describe:

POSSIBLE CAUSE / TRIGGER

☐ Loss of balance ☐ Freezing episode ☐ Fatigue

☐ Slippery surface ☐ Poor lighting ☐ Clutter / obstacle

☐ Medication wearing off Other: ____

INJURY DETAILS

☐ No injury ☐ Minor (bruises, soreness) ☐ Moderate (pain, swelling)
☐ Severe (possible fracture, head injury) **Body area affected:** _________

ASSISTANCE REQUIRED

☐ None ☐ Help from caregiver
☐ Medical attention needed Details: __________________________________

MEDICATION STATUS

- Medication taken on time? ☐ Yes ☐ No
- Time since last dose: ______________ Wearing-off noticed? ☐ Yes ☐ No

---

ENVIRONMENTAL FACTORS

☐ Poor lighting ☐ Wet/slippery floor ☐ Uneven surface ☐ Cluttered area

Other: ____

NOTES & OBSERVATIONS

What stood out about this incident?

INCIDENT SEVERITY RATING

☐ Low Risk ☐ Moderate Risk ☐ High Risk

PREVENTIVE ACTION (IMPORTANT)

What can be done to reduce future risk?

☐ Improve lighting
☐ Remove obstacles
☐ Adjust medication timing
☐ Increase supervision
☐ Use mobility aid

Other: ____

QUICK REMINDER

Every recorded fall helps build a clearer picture.
Patterns identified today can **prevent serious injuries tomorrow**.

FALL INCIDENT REPORT

Date: ____________________ **Time:** ____________________

LOCATION

Where did the fall occur?

☐ Bedroom ☐ Bathroom ☐ Living room ☐ Kitchen
☐ Outdoors ☐ Stairs Other: ________________________________

ACTIVITY AT THE TIME

What was the person doing?

☐ Walking ☐ Turning ☐ Standing up ☐ Sitting down
☐ Reaching for something ☐ Using stairs Other: __________

TYPE OF FALL

☐ Forward ☐ Backward ☐ Sideways ☐ Slipped
☐ Lost balance ☐ Unknown

WAS FREEZING INVOLVED?

☐ Yes ☐ No ☐ Unsure

If yes, describe:

POSSIBLE CAUSE / TRIGGER

☐ Loss of balance ☐ Freezing episode ☐ Fatigue

☐ Slippery surface ☐ Poor lighting ☐ Clutter / obstacle

☐ Medication wearing off Other: ____

INJURY DETAILS

☐ No injury ☐ Minor (bruises, soreness) ☐ Moderate (pain, swelling)
☐ Severe (possible fracture, head injury) **Body area affected:** _________

ASSISTANCE REQUIRED

☐ None ☐ Help from caregiver
☐ Medical attention needed Details: ___________________________________

MEDICATION STATUS

- Medication taken on time? ☐ Yes ☐ No
- Time since last dose: _______________ Wearing-off noticed? ☐ Yes ☐ No

---

ENVIRONMENTAL FACTORS

☐ Poor lighting ☐ Wet/slippery floor ☐ Uneven surface ☐ Cluttered area

Other: ____

NOTES & OBSERVATIONS

What stood out about this incident?

INCIDENT SEVERITY RATING

☐ Low Risk ☐ Moderate Risk ☐ High Risk

PREVENTIVE ACTION (IMPORTANT)

What can be done to reduce future risk?

☐ Improve lighting
☐ Remove obstacles
☐ Adjust medication timing
☐ Increase supervision
☐ Use mobility aid

Other: ____

QUICK REMINDER

Every recorded fall helps build a clearer picture.
Patterns identified today can **prevent serious injuries tomorrow**.

FALL INCIDENT REPORT

Date: ____________________ **Time:** ____________________

LOCATION

Where did the fall occur?

☐ Bedroom ☐ Bathroom ☐ Living room ☐ Kitchen
☐ Outdoors ☐ Stairs Other: ________________________________

ACTIVITY AT THE TIME

What was the person doing?

☐ Walking ☐ Turning ☐ Standing up ☐ Sitting down
☐ Reaching for something ☐ Using stairs Other: __________

TYPE OF FALL

☐ Forward ☐ Backward ☐ Sideways ☐ Slipped
☐ Lost balance ☐ Unknown

WAS FREEZING INVOLVED?

☐ Yes ☐ No ☐ Unsure

If yes, describe:

POSSIBLE CAUSE / TRIGGER

☐ Loss of balance ☐ Freezing episode ☐ Fatigue

☐ Slippery surface ☐ Poor lighting ☐ Clutter / obstacle

☐ Medication wearing off Other: ________________________________

INJURY DETAILS

☐ No injury ☐ Minor (bruises, soreness) ☐ Moderate (pain, swelling)
☐ Severe (possible fracture, head injury) **Body area affected:** _________

ASSISTANCE REQUIRED

☐ None ☐ Help from caregiver
☐ Medical attention needed Details: ___________________________________

MEDICATION STATUS

- Medication taken on time? ☐ Yes ☐ No
- Time since last dose: _______________ Wearing-off noticed? ☐ Yes ☐ No

---

ENVIRONMENTAL FACTORS

☐ Poor lighting ☐ Wet/slippery floor ☐ Uneven surface ☐ Cluttered area

Other: ____

NOTES & OBSERVATIONS

What stood out about this incident?

INCIDENT SEVERITY RATING

☐ Low Risk ☐ Moderate Risk ☐ High Risk

PREVENTIVE ACTION (IMPORTANT)

What can be done to reduce future risk?

☐ Improve lighting
☐ Remove obstacles
☐ Adjust medication timing
☐ Increase supervision
☐ Use mobility aid

Other: ____

QUICK REMINDER

Every recorded fall helps build a clearer picture.
Patterns identified today can **prevent serious injuries tomorrow**.

FALL INCIDENT REPORT

Date: ____________________ **Time:** ____________________

LOCATION

Where did the fall occur?

☐ Bedroom ☐ Bathroom ☐ Living room ☐ Kitchen
☐ Outdoors ☐ Stairs Other: ________________________________

ACTIVITY AT THE TIME

What was the person doing?

☐ Walking ☐ Turning ☐ Standing up ☐ Sitting down
☐ Reaching for something ☐ Using stairs Other: __________

TYPE OF FALL

☐ Forward ☐ Backward ☐ Sideways ☐ Slipped
☐ Lost balance ☐ Unknown

WAS FREEZING INVOLVED?

☐ Yes ☐ No ☐ Unsure

If yes, describe:

POSSIBLE CAUSE / TRIGGER

☐ Loss of balance ☐ Freezing episode ☐ Fatigue

☐ Slippery surface ☐ Poor lighting ☐ Clutter / obstacle

☐ Medication wearing off Other: ____________________________________

INJURY DETAILS

☐ No injury ☐ Minor (bruises, soreness) ☐ Moderate (pain, swelling)
☐ Severe (possible fracture, head injury) **Body area affected:** _________

ASSISTANCE REQUIRED

☐ None ☐ Help from caregiver
☐ Medical attention needed Details: ________________________________

MEDICATION STATUS

- Medication taken on time? ☐ Yes ☐ No
- Time since last dose: _______________ Wearing-off noticed? ☐ Yes ☐ No

---

ENVIRONMENTAL FACTORS

☐ Poor lighting ☐ Wet/slippery floor ☐ Uneven surface ☐ Cluttered area

Other: ____

NOTES & OBSERVATIONS

What stood out about this incident?

INCIDENT SEVERITY RATING

☐ Low Risk ☐ Moderate Risk ☐ High Risk

PREVENTIVE ACTION (IMPORTANT)

What can be done to reduce future risk?

☐ Improve lighting
☐ Remove obstacles
☐ Adjust medication timing
☐ Increase supervision
☐ Use mobility aid

Other: ____

QUICK REMINDER

Every recorded fall helps build a clearer picture.
Patterns identified today can **prevent serious injuries tomorrow**.

FALL INCIDENT REPORT

Date: ____________________ **Time:** ____________________

LOCATION

Where did the fall occur?

☐ Bedroom ☐ Bathroom ☐ Living room ☐ Kitchen
☐ Outdoors ☐ Stairs Other: ________________________________

ACTIVITY AT THE TIME

What was the person doing?

☐ Walking ☐ Turning ☐ Standing up ☐ Sitting down
☐ Reaching for something ☐ Using stairs Other: __________

TYPE OF FALL

☐ Forward ☐ Backward ☐ Sideways ☐ Slipped
☐ Lost balance ☐ Unknown

WAS FREEZING INVOLVED?

☐ Yes ☐ No ☐ Unsure

If yes, describe:

POSSIBLE CAUSE / TRIGGER

☐ Loss of balance ☐ Freezing episode ☐ Fatigue

☐ Slippery surface ☐ Poor lighting ☐ Clutter / obstacle

☐ Medication wearing off Other: ________________________________

INJURY DETAILS

☐ No injury ☐ Minor (bruises, soreness) ☐ Moderate (pain, swelling)
☐ Severe (possible fracture, head injury) **Body area affected:** _________

ASSISTANCE REQUIRED

☐ None ☐ Help from caregiver
☐ Medical attention needed Details: ________________________________

MEDICATION STATUS

- Medication taken on time? ☐ Yes ☐ No
- Time since last dose: _______________ Wearing-off noticed? ☐ Yes ☐ No

---

ENVIRONMENTAL FACTORS

☐ Poor lighting ☐ Wet/slippery floor ☐ Uneven surface ☐ Cluttered area

Other: ____

NOTES & OBSERVATIONS

What stood out about this incident?

INCIDENT SEVERITY RATING

☐ Low Risk ☐ Moderate Risk ☐ High Risk

PREVENTIVE ACTION (IMPORTANT)

What can be done to reduce future risk?

☐ Improve lighting
☐ Remove obstacles
☐ Adjust medication timing
☐ Increase supervision
☐ Use mobility aid

Other: ____

QUICK REMINDER

Every recorded fall helps build a clearer picture.
Patterns identified today can **prevent serious injuries tomorrow**.

FALL INCIDENT REPORT

Date: ____________________ **Time:** ____________________

LOCATION

Where did the fall occur?

☐ Bedroom ☐ Bathroom ☐ Living room ☐ Kitchen
☐ Outdoors ☐ Stairs Other: ________________________________

ACTIVITY AT THE TIME

What was the person doing?

☐ Walking ☐ Turning ☐ Standing up ☐ Sitting down
☐ Reaching for something ☐ Using stairs Other: __________

TYPE OF FALL

☐ Forward ☐ Backward ☐ Sideways ☐ Slipped
☐ Lost balance ☐ Unknown

WAS FREEZING INVOLVED?

☐ Yes ☐ No ☐ Unsure

If yes, describe:

POSSIBLE CAUSE / TRIGGER

☐ Loss of balance ☐ Freezing episode ☐ Fatigue

☐ Slippery surface ☐ Poor lighting ☐ Clutter / obstacle

☐ Medication wearing off Other: ____________________________________

INJURY DETAILS

☐ No injury ☐ Minor (bruises, soreness) ☐ Moderate (pain, swelling)
☐ Severe (possible fracture, head injury) **Body area affected:** _________

ASSISTANCE REQUIRED

☐ None ☐ Help from caregiver
☐ Medical attention needed Details: ________________________________

MEDICATION STATUS

- Medication taken on time? ☐ Yes ☐ No
- Time since last dose: _______________ Wearing-off noticed? ☐ Yes ☐ No

---

ENVIRONMENTAL FACTORS

☐ Poor lighting ☐ Wet/slippery floor ☐ Uneven surface ☐ Cluttered area

Other: ____

NOTES & OBSERVATIONS

What stood out about this incident?

INCIDENT SEVERITY RATING

☐ Low Risk ☐ Moderate Risk ☐ High Risk

PREVENTIVE ACTION (IMPORTANT)

What can be done to reduce future risk?

☐ Improve lighting
☐ Remove obstacles
☐ Adjust medication timing
☐ Increase supervision
☐ Use mobility aid

Other: ____

QUICK REMINDER

Every recorded fall helps build a clearer picture.
Patterns identified today can **prevent serious injuries tomorrow**.

FALL INCIDENT REPORT

Date: ____________________ **Time:** ____________________

LOCATION

Where did the fall occur?

☐ Bedroom ☐ Bathroom ☐ Living room ☐ Kitchen
☐ Outdoors ☐ Stairs Other: ________________________________

ACTIVITY AT THE TIME

What was the person doing?

☐ Walking ☐ Turning ☐ Standing up ☐ Sitting down
☐ Reaching for something ☐ Using stairs Other: __________

TYPE OF FALL

☐ Forward ☐ Backward ☐ Sideways ☐ Slipped
☐ Lost balance ☐ Unknown

WAS FREEZING INVOLVED?

☐ Yes ☐ No ☐ Unsure

If yes, describe:

POSSIBLE CAUSE / TRIGGER

☐ Loss of balance ☐ Freezing episode ☐ Fatigue

☐ Slippery surface ☐ Poor lighting ☐ Clutter / obstacle

☐ Medication wearing off Other: ____

INJURY DETAILS

☐ No injury ☐ Minor (bruises, soreness) ☐ Moderate (pain, swelling)
☐ Severe (possible fracture, head injury) **Body area affected:** _________

ASSISTANCE REQUIRED

☐ None ☐ Help from caregiver
☐ Medical attention needed Details: ___________________________________

MEDICATION STATUS

- Medication taken on time? ☐ Yes ☐ No
- Time since last dose: _______________ Wearing-off noticed? ☐ Yes ☐ No

---

ENVIRONMENTAL FACTORS

☐ Poor lighting ☐ Wet/slippery floor ☐ Uneven surface ☐ Cluttered area

Other: ____

NOTES & OBSERVATIONS

What stood out about this incident?

INCIDENT SEVERITY RATING

☐ Low Risk ☐ Moderate Risk ☐ High Risk

PREVENTIVE ACTION (IMPORTANT)

What can be done to reduce future risk?

☐ Improve lighting
☐ Remove obstacles
☐ Adjust medication timing
☐ Increase supervision
☐ Use mobility aid

Other: ____

QUICK REMINDER

Every recorded fall helps build a clearer picture.
Patterns identified today can **prevent serious injuries tomorrow**.

FALL INCIDENT REPORT

Date: ____________________ **Time:** ____________________

LOCATION

Where did the fall occur?

☐ Bedroom ☐ Bathroom ☐ Living room ☐ Kitchen
☐ Outdoors ☐ Stairs Other: ________________________________

ACTIVITY AT THE TIME

What was the person doing?

☐ Walking ☐ Turning ☐ Standing up ☐ Sitting down
☐ Reaching for something ☐ Using stairs Other: __________

TYPE OF FALL

☐ Forward ☐ Backward ☐ Sideways ☐ Slipped
☐ Lost balance ☐ Unknown

WAS FREEZING INVOLVED?

☐ Yes ☐ No ☐ Unsure

If yes, describe:

POSSIBLE CAUSE / TRIGGER

☐ Loss of balance ☐ Freezing episode ☐ Fatigue

☐ Slippery surface ☐ Poor lighting ☐ Clutter / obstacle

☐ Medication wearing off Other: ________________________________

INJURY DETAILS

☐ No injury ☐ Minor (bruises, soreness) ☐ Moderate (pain, swelling)
☐ Severe (possible fracture, head injury) **Body area affected:** _________

ASSISTANCE REQUIRED

☐ None ☐ Help from caregiver
☐ Medical attention needed Details: ___________________________________

MEDICATION STATUS

- Medication taken on time? ☐ Yes ☐ No
- Time since last dose: ______________ Wearing-off noticed? ☐ Yes ☐ No

---

ENVIRONMENTAL FACTORS

☐ Poor lighting ☐ Wet/slippery floor ☐ Uneven surface ☐ Cluttered area

Other: ____

NOTES & OBSERVATIONS

What stood out about this incident?

INCIDENT SEVERITY RATING

☐ Low Risk ☐ Moderate Risk ☐ High Risk

PREVENTIVE ACTION (IMPORTANT)

What can be done to reduce future risk?

☐ Improve lighting
☐ Remove obstacles
☐ Adjust medication timing
☐ Increase supervision
☐ Use mobility aid

Other: ____

QUICK REMINDER

Every recorded fall helps build a clearer picture.
Patterns identified today can **prevent serious injuries tomorrow**.

FALL INCIDENT REPORT

Date: ____________________ **Time:** ____________________

LOCATION

Where did the fall occur?

☐ Bedroom ☐ Bathroom ☐ Living room ☐ Kitchen
☐ Outdoors ☐ Stairs Other: ________________________________

ACTIVITY AT THE TIME

What was the person doing?

☐ Walking ☐ Turning ☐ Standing up ☐ Sitting down
☐ Reaching for something ☐ Using stairs Other: __________

TYPE OF FALL

☐ Forward ☐ Backward ☐ Sideways ☐ Slipped
☐ Lost balance ☐ Unknown

WAS FREEZING INVOLVED?

☐ Yes ☐ No ☐ Unsure

If yes, describe:

POSSIBLE CAUSE / TRIGGER

☐ Loss of balance ☐ Freezing episode ☐ Fatigue

☐ Slippery surface ☐ Poor lighting ☐ Clutter / obstacle

☐ Medication wearing off Other: ____

INJURY DETAILS

☐ No injury ☐ Minor (bruises, soreness) ☐ Moderate (pain, swelling)
☐ Severe (possible fracture, head injury) **Body area affected:** _________

ASSISTANCE REQUIRED

☐ None ☐ Help from caregiver
☐ Medical attention needed Details: ___________________________________

MEDICATION STATUS

- Medication taken on time? ☐ Yes ☐ No
- Time since last dose: _______________ Wearing-off noticed? ☐ Yes ☐ No

---

ENVIRONMENTAL FACTORS

☐ Poor lighting ☐ Wet/slippery floor ☐ Uneven surface ☐ Cluttered area

Other: ____

NOTES & OBSERVATIONS

What stood out about this incident?

INCIDENT SEVERITY RATING

☐ Low Risk ☐ Moderate Risk ☐ High Risk

PREVENTIVE ACTION (IMPORTANT)

What can be done to reduce future risk?

☐ Improve lighting
☐ Remove obstacles
☐ Adjust medication timing
☐ Increase supervision
☐ Use mobility aid

Other: ____

QUICK REMINDER

Every recorded fall helps build a clearer picture.
Patterns identified today can **prevent serious injuries tomorrow**.

Section 3 - Freezing Episode Tracker

(Detailed Monitoring for Safety & Prevention)

Purpose of This Section

Freezing episodes can happen suddenly and are a major cause of falls in Parkinson's disease.

Tracking each episode helps you:

- Identify **common triggers**
- Understand **when and where freezing occurs**
- Reduce risk through **better planning and prevention**
- Record every episode of freezing when it happens
- Use this page whenever a freezing episode occurs

FREEZING EPISODE LOG

Date: ____________________ **Time:** ____________________

LOCATION

Where did the freezing occur?

☐ Bedroom ☐ Bathroom ☐ Living room ☐ Hallway/doorway
☐ Kitchen ☐ Outdoors Other: ________________________________

ACTIVITY AT THE TIME

What was the person doing?

☐ Starting to walk ☐ Turning / changing direction ☐ Walking through doorway
☐ Stopping suddenly ☐ Walking in crowded space Other: _________________

DURATION OF EPISODE

☐ Less than 10 seconds ☐ 10–30 seconds
☐ 30–60 seconds ☐ More than 1 minute

SEVERITY LEVEL

☐ Mild (brief pause, quickly resumed)
☐ Moderate (needed time or cue to move)
☐ Severe (unable to move without assistance)

ASSISTANCE REQUIRED

☐ None ☐ Verbal cue ☐ Physical assistance Details: _______________

POSSIBLE TRIGGER

☐ Turning ☐ Doorway / narrow space ☐ Stress or anxiety ☐ Fatigue
☐ Distraction ☐ Medication wearing off Other: __________________________

DID A FALL OR NEAR-FALL OCCUR?

☐ No ☐ Near-fall ☐ Fall

If yes, describe:

MEDICATION STATUS

- Medication taken on time? ☐ Yes ☐ No
- Time since last dose: __________Wearing-off symptoms noticed? ☐ Yes ☐ No

ENVIRONMENTAL FACTORS

☐ Poor lighting ☐ Cluttered space ☐ Uneven surface

☐ Noise / distractions Other: ______________________________________

NOTES & OBSERVATIONS

What stood out about this episode?

EPISODE IMPACT RATING

☐ Low Impact

☐ Moderate Impact

☐ High Impact

PREVENTIVE ACTION

What may help prevent this in the future?

☐ Slow down movements

☐ Use verbal cueing (counting, rhythm)

☐ Improve environment (lighting, space)

☐ Adjust medication timing

☐ Provide supervision

Other: ______________________________________

QUICK REMINDER

Freezing episodes often follow patterns.
Tracking them consistently helps you **anticipate and prevent risk**.

FREEZING EPISODE LOG

Date: ____________________ **Time:** ____________________

LOCATION

Where did the freezing occur?

☐ Bedroom ☐ Bathroom ☐ Living room ☐ Hallway/doorway
☐ Kitchen ☐ Outdoors Other: ________________________________

ACTIVITY AT THE TIME

What was the person doing?

☐ Starting to walk ☐ Turning / changing direction ☐ Walking through doorway
☐ Stopping suddenly ☐ Walking in crowded space Other: _________________

DURATION OF EPISODE

☐ Less than 10 seconds ☐ 10–30 seconds
☐ 30–60 seconds ☐ More than 1 minute

SEVERITY LEVEL

☐ Mild (brief pause, quickly resumed)
☐ Moderate (needed time or cue to move)
☐ Severe (unable to move without assistance)

ASSISTANCE REQUIRED

☐ None ☐ Verbal cue ☐ Physical assistance Details: _______________

POSSIBLE TRIGGER

☐ Turning ☐ Doorway / narrow space ☐ Stress or anxiety ☐ Fatigue
☐ Distraction ☐ Medication wearing off Other: __________________________

DID A FALL OR NEAR-FALL OCCUR?

☐ No ☐ Near-fall ☐ Fall

If yes, describe:

MEDICATION STATUS

- Medication taken on time? ☐ Yes ☐ No
- Time since last dose: __________Wearing-off symptoms noticed? ☐ Yes ☐ No

ENVIRONMENTAL FACTORS

☐ Poor lighting ☐ Cluttered space ☐ Uneven surface
☐ Noise / distractions Other: ____

NOTES & OBSERVATIONS

What stood out about this episode?

EPISODE IMPACT RATING

☐ Low Impact
☐ Moderate Impact
☐ High Impact

PREVENTIVE ACTION

What may help prevent this in the future?

☐ Slow down movements
☐ Use verbal cueing (counting, rhythm)
☐ Improve environment (lighting, space)
☐ Adjust medication timing
☐ Provide supervision

Other: ____

QUICK REMINDER

Freezing episodes often follow patterns.
Tracking them consistently helps you **anticipate and prevent risk**.

FREEZING EPISODE LOG

Date: ____________________ **Time:** ____________________

LOCATION

Where did the freezing occur?

☐ Bedroom ☐ Bathroom ☐ Living room ☐ Hallway/doorway
☐ Kitchen ☐ Outdoors Other: ________________________________

ACTIVITY AT THE TIME

What was the person doing?

☐ Starting to walk ☐ Turning / changing direction ☐ Walking through doorway
☐ Stopping suddenly ☐ Walking in crowded space Other: _________________

DURATION OF EPISODE

☐ Less than 10 seconds ☐ 10–30 seconds
☐ 30–60 seconds ☐ More than 1 minute

SEVERITY LEVEL

☐ Mild (brief pause, quickly resumed)
☐ Moderate (needed time or cue to move)
☐ Severe (unable to move without assistance)

ASSISTANCE REQUIRED

☐ None ☐ Verbal cue ☐ Physical assistance Details: _______________

POSSIBLE TRIGGER

☐ Turning ☐ Doorway / narrow space ☐ Stress or anxiety ☐ Fatigue
☐ Distraction ☐ Medication wearing off Other: __________________________

DID A FALL OR NEAR-FALL OCCUR?

☐ No ☐ Near-fall ☐ Fall

If yes, describe:

MEDICATION STATUS

- Medication taken on time? ☐ Yes ☐ No
- Time since last dose: __________Wearing-off symptoms noticed? ☐ Yes ☐ No

ENVIRONMENTAL FACTORS

☐ Poor lighting ☐ Cluttered space ☐ Uneven surface
☐ Noise / distractions Other: ____

NOTES & OBSERVATIONS

What stood out about this episode?

EPISODE IMPACT RATING

☐ Low Impact
☐ Moderate Impact
☐ High Impact

PREVENTIVE ACTION

What may help prevent this in the future?

☐ Slow down movements
☐ Use verbal cueing (counting, rhythm)
☐ Improve environment (lighting, space)
☐ Adjust medication timing
☐ Provide supervision

Other: ____

QUICK REMINDER

Freezing episodes often follow patterns.
Tracking them consistently helps you **anticipate and prevent risk**.

FREEZING EPISODE LOG

Date: ____________________ **Time:** ____________________

LOCATION

Where did the freezing occur?

☐ Bedroom ☐ Bathroom ☐ Living room ☐ Hallway/doorway
☐ Kitchen ☐ Outdoors Other: ________________________________

ACTIVITY AT THE TIME

What was the person doing?

☐ Starting to walk ☐ Turning / changing direction ☐ Walking through doorway
☐ Stopping suddenly ☐ Walking in crowded space Other: ________________

DURATION OF EPISODE

☐ Less than 10 seconds ☐ 10–30 seconds
☐ 30–60 seconds ☐ More than 1 minute

SEVERITY LEVEL

☐ Mild (brief pause, quickly resumed)
☐ Moderate (needed time or cue to move)
☐ Severe (unable to move without assistance)

ASSISTANCE REQUIRED

☐ None ☐ Verbal cue ☐ Physical assistance Details: _______________

POSSIBLE TRIGGER

☐ Turning ☐ Doorway / narrow space ☐ Stress or anxiety ☐ Fatigue
☐ Distraction ☐ Medication wearing off Other: __________________________

DID A FALL OR NEAR-FALL OCCUR?

☐ No ☐ Near-fall ☐ Fall

If yes, describe:

MEDICATION STATUS

- Medication taken on time? ☐ Yes ☐ No
- Time since last dose: __________ Wearing-off symptoms noticed? ☐ Yes ☐ No

ENVIRONMENTAL FACTORS

☐ Poor lighting ☐ Cluttered space ☐ Uneven surface
☐ Noise / distractions Other: ____

NOTES & OBSERVATIONS

What stood out about this episode?

EPISODE IMPACT RATING

☐ Low Impact
☐ Moderate Impact
☐ High Impact

PREVENTIVE ACTION

What may help prevent this in the future?

☐ Slow down movements
☐ Use verbal cueing (counting, rhythm)
☐ Improve environment (lighting, space)
☐ Adjust medication timing
☐ Provide supervision

Other: ____

QUICK REMINDER

Freezing episodes often follow patterns.
Tracking them consistently helps you **anticipate and prevent risk**.

FREEZING EPISODE LOG

Date: ____________________ **Time:** ____________________

LOCATION

Where did the freezing occur?

☐ Bedroom ☐ Bathroom ☐ Living room ☐ Hallway/doorway
☐ Kitchen ☐ Outdoors Other: ________________________________

ACTIVITY AT THE TIME

What was the person doing?

☐ Starting to walk ☐ Turning / changing direction ☐ Walking through doorway
☐ Stopping suddenly ☐ Walking in crowded space Other: _________________

DURATION OF EPISODE

☐ Less than 10 seconds ☐ 10–30 seconds
☐ 30–60 seconds ☐ More than 1 minute

SEVERITY LEVEL

☐ Mild (brief pause, quickly resumed)
☐ Moderate (needed time or cue to move)
☐ Severe (unable to move without assistance)

ASSISTANCE REQUIRED

☐ None ☐ Verbal cue ☐ Physical assistance Details: _______________

POSSIBLE TRIGGER

☐ Turning ☐ Doorway / narrow space ☐ Stress or anxiety ☐ Fatigue
☐ Distraction ☐ Medication wearing off Other: __________________________

DID A FALL OR NEAR-FALL OCCUR?

☐ No ☐ Near-fall ☐ Fall

If yes, describe:

MEDICATION STATUS

- Medication taken on time? ☐ Yes ☐ No
- Time since last dose: __________ Wearing-off symptoms noticed? ☐ Yes ☐ No

ENVIRONMENTAL FACTORS

☐ Poor lighting ☐ Cluttered space ☐ Uneven surface
☐ Noise / distractions Other: ______________________________

NOTES & OBSERVATIONS

What stood out about this episode?

EPISODE IMPACT RATING

☐ Low Impact
☐ Moderate Impact
☐ High Impact

PREVENTIVE ACTION

What may help prevent this in the future?

☐ Slow down movements
☐ Use verbal cueing (counting, rhythm)
☐ Improve environment (lighting, space)
☐ Adjust medication timing
☐ Provide supervision

Other: ______________________________

QUICK REMINDER

Freezing episodes often follow patterns.
Tracking them consistently helps you **anticipate and prevent risk**.

FREEZING EPISODE LOG

Date: ____________________ **Time:** ____________________

LOCATION

Where did the freezing occur?

☐ Bedroom ☐ Bathroom ☐ Living room ☐ Hallway/doorway
☐ Kitchen ☐ Outdoors Other: ________________________________

ACTIVITY AT THE TIME

What was the person doing?

☐ Starting to walk ☐ Turning / changing direction ☐ Walking through doorway
☐ Stopping suddenly ☐ Walking in crowded space Other: __________________

DURATION OF EPISODE

☐ Less than 10 seconds ☐ 10–30 seconds
☐ 30–60 seconds ☐ More than 1 minute

SEVERITY LEVEL

☐ Mild (brief pause, quickly resumed)
☐ Moderate (needed time or cue to move)
☐ Severe (unable to move without assistance)

ASSISTANCE REQUIRED

☐ None ☐ Verbal cue ☐ Physical assistance Details: _______________

POSSIBLE TRIGGER

☐ Turning ☐ Doorway / narrow space ☐ Stress or anxiety ☐ Fatigue
☐ Distraction ☐ Medication wearing off Other: __________________________

DID A FALL OR NEAR-FALL OCCUR?

☐ No ☐ Near-fall ☐ Fall

If yes, describe:

MEDICATION STATUS

- Medication taken on time? ☐ Yes ☐ No
- Time since last dose: __________Wearing-off symptoms noticed? ☐ Yes ☐ No

ENVIRONMENTAL FACTORS

☐ Poor lighting ☐ Cluttered space ☐ Uneven surface
☐ Noise / distractions Other: ______________________________

NOTES & OBSERVATIONS

What stood out about this episode?

EPISODE IMPACT RATING

☐ Low Impact
☐ Moderate Impact
☐ High Impact

PREVENTIVE ACTION

What may help prevent this in the future?

☐ Slow down movements
☐ Use verbal cueing (counting, rhythm)
☐ Improve environment (lighting, space)
☐ Adjust medication timing
☐ Provide supervision

Other: ______________________________

QUICK REMINDER

Freezing episodes often follow patterns.
Tracking them consistently helps you **anticipate and prevent risk**.

FREEZING EPISODE LOG

Date: ____________________ **Time:** ____________________

LOCATION

Where did the freezing occur?

☐ Bedroom ☐ Bathroom ☐ Living room ☐ Hallway/doorway
☐ Kitchen ☐ Outdoors Other: ________________________________

ACTIVITY AT THE TIME

What was the person doing?

☐ Starting to walk ☐ Turning / changing direction ☐ Walking through doorway
☐ Stopping suddenly ☐ Walking in crowded space Other: _________________

DURATION OF EPISODE

☐ Less than 10 seconds ☐ 10–30 seconds
☐ 30–60 seconds ☐ More than 1 minute

SEVERITY LEVEL

☐ Mild (brief pause, quickly resumed)
☐ Moderate (needed time or cue to move)
☐ Severe (unable to move without assistance)

ASSISTANCE REQUIRED

☐ None ☐ Verbal cue ☐ Physical assistance Details: _______________

POSSIBLE TRIGGER

☐ Turning ☐ Doorway / narrow space ☐ Stress or anxiety ☐ Fatigue
☐ Distraction ☐ Medication wearing off Other: __________________________

DID A FALL OR NEAR-FALL OCCUR?

☐ No ☐ Near-fall ☐ Fall

If yes, describe:

MEDICATION STATUS

- Medication taken on time? ☐ Yes ☐ No
- Time since last dose: __________Wearing-off symptoms noticed? ☐ Yes ☐ No

ENVIRONMENTAL FACTORS

☐ Poor lighting ☐ Cluttered space ☐ Uneven surface
☐ Noise / distractions Other: ____

NOTES & OBSERVATIONS

What stood out about this episode?

EPISODE IMPACT RATING

☐ Low Impact
☐ Moderate Impact
☐ High Impact

PREVENTIVE ACTION

What may help prevent this in the future?

☐ Slow down movements
☐ Use verbal cueing (counting, rhythm)
☐ Improve environment (lighting, space)
☐ Adjust medication timing
☐ Provide supervision

Other: ____

QUICK REMINDER

Freezing episodes often follow patterns.
Tracking them consistently helps you **anticipate and prevent risk**.

FREEZING EPISODE LOG

Date: ____________________ **Time:** ____________________

LOCATION

Where did the freezing occur?

☐ Bedroom ☐ Bathroom ☐ Living room ☐ Hallway/doorway
☐ Kitchen ☐ Outdoors Other: ________________________________

ACTIVITY AT THE TIME

What was the person doing?

☐ Starting to walk ☐ Turning / changing direction ☐ Walking through doorway
☐ Stopping suddenly ☐ Walking in crowded space Other: __________________

DURATION OF EPISODE

☐ Less than 10 seconds ☐ 10–30 seconds
☐ 30–60 seconds ☐ More than 1 minute

SEVERITY LEVEL

☐ Mild (brief pause, quickly resumed)
☐ Moderate (needed time or cue to move)
☐ Severe (unable to move without assistance)

ASSISTANCE REQUIRED

☐ None ☐ Verbal cue ☐ Physical assistance Details: _______________

POSSIBLE TRIGGER

☐ Turning ☐ Doorway / narrow space ☐ Stress or anxiety ☐ Fatigue
☐ Distraction ☐ Medication wearing off Other: __________________________

DID A FALL OR NEAR-FALL OCCUR?

☐ No ☐ Near-fall ☐ Fall

If yes, describe:

MEDICATION STATUS

- Medication taken on time? ☐ Yes ☐ No
- Time since last dose: __________Wearing-off symptoms noticed? ☐ Yes ☐ No

ENVIRONMENTAL FACTORS

☐ Poor lighting ☐ Cluttered space ☐ Uneven surface
☐ Noise / distractions Other: ____

NOTES & OBSERVATIONS

What stood out about this episode?

EPISODE IMPACT RATING

☐ Low Impact
☐ Moderate Impact
☐ High Impact

PREVENTIVE ACTION

What may help prevent this in the future?

☐ Slow down movements
☐ Use verbal cueing (counting, rhythm)
☐ Improve environment (lighting, space)
☐ Adjust medication timing
☐ Provide supervision

Other: ____

QUICK REMINDER

Freezing episodes often follow patterns.
Tracking them consistently helps you **anticipate and prevent risk**.

FREEZING EPISODE LOG

Date: ____________________ **Time:** ____________________

LOCATION

Where did the freezing occur?

☐ Bedroom ☐ Bathroom ☐ Living room ☐ Hallway/doorway
☐ Kitchen ☐ Outdoors Other: ________________________________

ACTIVITY AT THE TIME

What was the person doing?

☐ Starting to walk ☐ Turning / changing direction ☐ Walking through doorway
☐ Stopping suddenly ☐ Walking in crowded space Other: _________________

DURATION OF EPISODE

☐ Less than 10 seconds ☐ 10–30 seconds
☐ 30–60 seconds ☐ More than 1 minute

SEVERITY LEVEL

☐ Mild (brief pause, quickly resumed)
☐ Moderate (needed time or cue to move)
☐ Severe (unable to move without assistance)

ASSISTANCE REQUIRED

☐ None ☐ Verbal cue ☐ Physical assistance Details: _______________

POSSIBLE TRIGGER

☐ Turning ☐ Doorway / narrow space ☐ Stress or anxiety ☐ Fatigue
☐ Distraction ☐ Medication wearing off Other: __________________________

DID A FALL OR NEAR-FALL OCCUR?

☐ No ☐ Near-fall ☐ Fall

If yes, describe:

MEDICATION STATUS

- Medication taken on time? ☐ Yes ☐ No
- Time since last dose: __________Wearing-off symptoms noticed? ☐ Yes ☐ No

ENVIRONMENTAL FACTORS

☐ Poor lighting ☐ Cluttered space ☐ Uneven surface
☐ Noise / distractions Other: ____

NOTES & OBSERVATIONS

What stood out about this episode?

EPISODE IMPACT RATING

☐ Low Impact
☐ Moderate Impact
☐ High Impact

PREVENTIVE ACTION

What may help prevent this in the future?

☐ Slow down movements
☐ Use verbal cueing (counting, rhythm)
☐ Improve environment (lighting, space)
☐ Adjust medication timing
☐ Provide supervision

Other: ____

QUICK REMINDER

Freezing episodes often follow patterns.
Tracking them consistently helps you **anticipate and prevent risk**.

FREEZING EPISODE LOG

Date: ____________________ **Time:** ____________________

LOCATION

Where did the freezing occur?

☐ Bedroom ☐ Bathroom ☐ Living room ☐ Hallway/doorway
☐ Kitchen ☐ Outdoors Other: ________________________________

ACTIVITY AT THE TIME

What was the person doing?

☐ Starting to walk ☐ Turning / changing direction ☐ Walking through doorway
☐ Stopping suddenly ☐ Walking in crowded space Other: _________________

DURATION OF EPISODE

☐ Less than 10 seconds ☐ 10–30 seconds
☐ 30–60 seconds ☐ More than 1 minute

SEVERITY LEVEL

☐ Mild (brief pause, quickly resumed)
☐ Moderate (needed time or cue to move)
☐ Severe (unable to move without assistance)

ASSISTANCE REQUIRED

☐ None ☐ Verbal cue ☐ Physical assistance Details: _______________

POSSIBLE TRIGGER

☐ Turning ☐ Doorway / narrow space ☐ Stress or anxiety ☐ Fatigue
☐ Distraction ☐ Medication wearing off Other: __________________________

DID A FALL OR NEAR-FALL OCCUR?

☐ No ☐ Near-fall ☐ Fall

If yes, describe:

MEDICATION STATUS

- Medication taken on time? ☐ Yes ☐ No
- Time since last dose: __________Wearing-off symptoms noticed? ☐ Yes ☐ No

ENVIRONMENTAL FACTORS

☐ Poor lighting ☐ Cluttered space ☐ Uneven surface
☐ Noise / distractions Other: ____________________________________

NOTES & OBSERVATIONS

What stood out about this episode?

EPISODE IMPACT RATING

☐ Low Impact
☐ Moderate Impact
☐ High Impact

PREVENTIVE ACTION

What may help prevent this in the future?

☐ Slow down movements
☐ Use verbal cueing (counting, rhythm)
☐ Improve environment (lighting, space)
☐ Adjust medication timing
☐ Provide supervision

Other: ______________________________________

QUICK REMINDER

Freezing episodes often follow patterns.
Tracking them consistently helps you **anticipate and prevent risk**.

FREEZING EPISODE LOG

Date: ____________________ **Time:** ____________________

LOCATION

Where did the freezing occur?

☐ Bedroom ☐ Bathroom ☐ Living room ☐ Hallway/doorway
☐ Kitchen ☐ Outdoors Other: ________________________________

ACTIVITY AT THE TIME

What was the person doing?

☐ Starting to walk ☐ Turning / changing direction ☐ Walking through doorway
☐ Stopping suddenly ☐ Walking in crowded space Other: _________________

DURATION OF EPISODE

☐ Less than 10 seconds ☐ 10–30 seconds
☐ 30–60 seconds ☐ More than 1 minute

SEVERITY LEVEL

☐ Mild (brief pause, quickly resumed)
☐ Moderate (needed time or cue to move)
☐ Severe (unable to move without assistance)

ASSISTANCE REQUIRED

☐ None ☐ Verbal cue ☐ Physical assistance Details: _______________

POSSIBLE TRIGGER

☐ Turning ☐ Doorway / narrow space ☐ Stress or anxiety ☐ Fatigue
☐ Distraction ☐ Medication wearing off Other: __________________________

DID A FALL OR NEAR-FALL OCCUR?

☐ No ☐ Near-fall ☐ Fall

If yes, describe:

MEDICATION STATUS

- Medication taken on time? ☐ Yes ☐ No
- Time since last dose: __________Wearing-off symptoms noticed? ☐ Yes ☐ No

ENVIRONMENTAL FACTORS

☐ Poor lighting ☐ Cluttered space ☐ Uneven surface
☐ Noise / distractions Other: ______________________________

NOTES & OBSERVATIONS

What stood out about this episode?

EPISODE IMPACT RATING

☐ Low Impact
☐ Moderate Impact
☐ High Impact

PREVENTIVE ACTION

What may help prevent this in the future?

☐ Slow down movements
☐ Use verbal cueing (counting, rhythm)
☐ Improve environment (lighting, space)
☐ Adjust medication timing
☐ Provide supervision

Other: ______________________________

QUICK REMINDER

Freezing episodes often follow patterns.
Tracking them consistently helps you **anticipate and prevent risk**.

FREEZING EPISODE LOG

Date: ____________________ **Time:** ____________________

LOCATION

Where did the freezing occur?

☐ Bedroom ☐ Bathroom ☐ Living room ☐ Hallway/doorway
☐ Kitchen ☐ Outdoors Other: ________________________________

ACTIVITY AT THE TIME

What was the person doing?

☐ Starting to walk ☐ Turning / changing direction ☐ Walking through doorway
☐ Stopping suddenly ☐ Walking in crowded space Other: _________________

DURATION OF EPISODE

☐ Less than 10 seconds ☐ 10–30 seconds
☐ 30–60 seconds ☐ More than 1 minute

SEVERITY LEVEL

☐ Mild (brief pause, quickly resumed)
☐ Moderate (needed time or cue to move)
☐ Severe (unable to move without assistance)

ASSISTANCE REQUIRED

☐ None ☐ Verbal cue ☐ Physical assistance Details: _______________

POSSIBLE TRIGGER

☐ Turning ☐ Doorway / narrow space ☐ Stress or anxiety ☐ Fatigue
☐ Distraction ☐ Medication wearing off Other: ___________________________

DID A FALL OR NEAR-FALL OCCUR?

☐ No ☐ Near-fall ☐ Fall

If yes, describe:

MEDICATION STATUS

- Medication taken on time? ☐ Yes ☐ No
- Time since last dose: ___________Wearing-off symptoms noticed? ☐ Yes ☐ No

ENVIRONMENTAL FACTORS

☐ Poor lighting ☐ Cluttered space ☐ Uneven surface

☐ Noise / distractions Other: ______________________________

NOTES & OBSERVATIONS

What stood out about this episode?

EPISODE IMPACT RATING

☐ Low Impact

☐ Moderate Impact

☐ High Impact

PREVENTIVE ACTION

What may help prevent this in the future?

☐ Slow down movements

☐ Use verbal cueing (counting, rhythm)

☐ Improve environment (lighting, space)

☐ Adjust medication timing

☐ Provide supervision

Other: ______________________________

QUICK REMINDER

Freezing episodes often follow patterns.
Tracking them consistently helps you **anticipate and prevent risk**.

Section 4 - Daily Safety Check & Risk Rating

(Quick Daily Monitoring for Fall & Freezing Risk)

Purpose of This Section

Not every risk leads to a fall or freezing episode—but daily monitoring helps you **identify warning signs early**.

This quick check takes just **1–2 minutes** and helps you:

- Stay aware of daily risks
- Track subtle changes
- Prevent incidents before they happen
- Complete once daily for best results.

DAILY SAFETY CHECK **Date: ______________** **Day : ____ of 90**

- Any freezing today? ☐ Yes ☐ No
- Any falls today? ☐ Yes ☐ No

Risk Factors Observed

☐ Fatigue
☐ Medication wearing off
☐ Environmental hazards

Overall Safety Rating

☐ Safe ☐ Caution ☐ High Risk

Notes

DAILY SAFETY CHECK **Date: ______________** **Day : ____ of 90**

- Any freezing today? ☐ Yes ☐ No
- Any falls today? ☐ Yes ☐ No

Risk Factors Observed

☐ Fatigue
☐ Medication wearing off
☐ Environmental hazards

Overall Safety Rating

☐ Safe ☐ Caution ☐ High Risk

Notes

.DAILY SAFETY CHECK **Date: ________________** **Day : ____ of 90**

- Any freezing today? ☐ Yes ☐ No
- Any falls today? ☐ Yes ☐ No

Risk Factors Observed

☐ Fatigue
☐ Medication wearing off
☐ Environmental hazards

Overall Safety Rating

☐ Safe ☐ Caution ☐ High Risk

Notes

DAILY SAFETY CHECK **Date: ________________** **Day : ____ of 90**

- Any freezing today? ☐ Yes ☐ No
- Any falls today? ☐ Yes ☐ No

Risk Factors Observed

☐ Fatigue
☐ Medication wearing off
☐ Environmental hazards

Overall Safety Rating

☐ Safe ☐ Caution ☐ High Risk

Notes

.DAILY SAFETY CHECK Date: ______________ Day : ____ of 90

- Any freezing today? ☐ Yes ☐ No
- Any falls today? ☐ Yes ☐ No

Risk Factors Observed

☐ Fatigue
☐ Medication wearing off
☐ Environmental hazards

Overall Safety Rating

☐ Safe ☐ Caution ☐ High Risk

Notes

DAILY SAFETY CHECK Date: ______________ Day : ____ of 90

- Any freezing today? ☐ Yes ☐ No
- Any falls today? ☐ Yes ☐ No

Risk Factors Observed

☐ Fatigue
☐ Medication wearing off
☐ Environmental hazards

Overall Safety Rating

☐ Safe ☐ Caution ☐ High Risk

Notes

.DAILY SAFETY CHECK **Date:** ______________ **Day : ____ of 90**

- Any freezing today? ☐ Yes ☐ No
- Any falls today? ☐ Yes ☐ No

Risk Factors Observed

☐ Fatigue
☐ Medication wearing off
☐ Environmental hazards

Overall Safety Rating

☐ Safe ☐ Caution ☐ High Risk

Notes

DAILY SAFETY CHECK **Date:** ______________ **Day : ____ of 90**

- Any freezing today? ☐ Yes ☐ No
- Any falls today? ☐ Yes ☐ No

Risk Factors Observed

☐ Fatigue
☐ Medication wearing off
☐ Environmental hazards

Overall Safety Rating

☐ Safe ☐ Caution ☐ High Risk

Notes

.DAILY SAFETY CHECK Date: _______________ Day : ____ of 90

- Any freezing today? ☐ Yes ☐ No
- Any falls today? ☐ Yes ☐ No

Risk Factors Observed

☐ Fatigue
☐ Medication wearing off
☐ Environmental hazards

Overall Safety Rating

☐ Safe ☐ Caution ☐ High Risk

Notes

DAILY SAFETY CHECK Date: _______________ Day : ____ of 90

- Any freezing today? ☐ Yes ☐ No
- Any falls today? ☐ Yes ☐ No

Risk Factors Observed

☐ Fatigue
☐ Medication wearing off
☐ Environmental hazards

Overall Safety Rating

☐ Safe ☐ Caution ☐ High Risk

Notes

.DAILY SAFETY CHECK Date: ______________ Day : ____ of 90

- Any freezing today? ☐ Yes ☐ No
- Any falls today? ☐ Yes ☐ No

Risk Factors Observed

☐ Fatigue
☐ Medication wearing off
☐ Environmental hazards

Overall Safety Rating

☐ Safe ☐ Caution ☐ High Risk

Notes

DAILY SAFETY CHECK Date: ______________ Day : ____ of 90

- Any freezing today? ☐ Yes ☐ No
- Any falls today? ☐ Yes ☐ No

Risk Factors Observed

☐ Fatigue
☐ Medication wearing off
☐ Environmental hazards

Overall Safety Rating

☐ Safe ☐ Caution ☐ High Risk

Notes

.DAILY SAFETY CHECK Date: _______________ Day : ____ of 90

- Any freezing today? ☐ Yes ☐ No
- Any falls today? ☐ Yes ☐ No

Risk Factors Observed

☐ Fatigue
☐ Medication wearing off
☐ Environmental hazards

Overall Safety Rating

☐ Safe ☐ Caution ☐ High Risk

Notes

DAILY SAFETY CHECK Date: _______________ Day : ____ of 90

- Any freezing today? ☐ Yes ☐ No
- Any falls today? ☐ Yes ☐ No

Risk Factors Observed

☐ Fatigue
☐ Medication wearing off
☐ Environmental hazards

Overall Safety Rating

☐ Safe ☐ Caution ☐ High Risk

Notes

.DAILY SAFETY CHECK Date: ______________ Day : ____ of 90

- Any freezing today? ☐ Yes ☐ No
- Any falls today? ☐ Yes ☐ No

Risk Factors Observed

☐ Fatigue
☐ Medication wearing off
☐ Environmental hazards

Overall Safety Rating

☐ Safe ☐ Caution ☐ High Risk

Notes

DAILY SAFETY CHECK Date: ______________ Day : ____ of 90

- Any freezing today? ☐ Yes ☐ No
- Any falls today? ☐ Yes ☐ No

Risk Factors Observed

☐ Fatigue
☐ Medication wearing off
☐ Environmental hazards

Overall Safety Rating

☐ Safe ☐ Caution ☐ High Risk

Notes

.**DAILY SAFETY CHECK** **Date:** ________________ **Day :** ____ **of 90**

- Any freezing today? ☐ Yes ☐ No
- Any falls today? ☐ Yes ☐ No

Risk Factors Observed

☐ Fatigue
☐ Medication wearing off
☐ Environmental hazards

Overall Safety Rating

☐ Safe ☐ Caution ☐ High Risk

Notes

DAILY SAFETY CHECK **Date:** ________________ **Day :** ____ **of 90**

- Any freezing today? ☐ Yes ☐ No
- Any falls today? ☐ Yes ☐ No

Risk Factors Observed

☐ Fatigue
☐ Medication wearing off
☐ Environmental hazards

Overall Safety Rating

☐ Safe ☐ Caution ☐ High Risk

Notes

.DAILY SAFETY CHECK Date: ______________ Day : ____ of 90

- Any freezing today? ☐ Yes ☐ No
- Any falls today? ☐ Yes ☐ No

Risk Factors Observed

☐ Fatigue
☐ Medication wearing off
☐ Environmental hazards

Overall Safety Rating

☐ Safe ☐ Caution ☐ High Risk

Notes

DAILY SAFETY CHECK Date: ______________ Day : ____ of 90

- Any freezing today? ☐ Yes ☐ No
- Any falls today? ☐ Yes ☐ No

Risk Factors Observed

☐ Fatigue
☐ Medication wearing off
☐ Environmental hazards

Overall Safety Rating

☐ Safe ☐ Caution ☐ High Risk

Notes

.DAILY SAFETY CHECK **Date: ________________** **Day : ____ of 90**

- Any freezing today? ☐ Yes ☐ No
- Any falls today? ☐ Yes ☐ No

Risk Factors Observed

☐ Fatigue
☐ Medication wearing off
☐ Environmental hazards

Overall Safety Rating

☐ Safe ☐ Caution ☐ High Risk

Notes

DAILY SAFETY CHECK **Date: ________________** **Day : ____ of 90**

- Any freezing today? ☐ Yes ☐ No
- Any falls today? ☐ Yes ☐ No

Risk Factors Observed

☐ Fatigue
☐ Medication wearing off
☐ Environmental hazards

Overall Safety Rating

☐ Safe ☐ Caution ☐ High Risk

Notes

.DAILY SAFETY CHECK **Date: ________________** **Day : ____ of 90**

- Any freezing today? ☐ Yes ☐ No
- Any falls today? ☐ Yes ☐ No

Risk Factors Observed

☐ Fatigue
☐ Medication wearing off
☐ Environmental hazards

Overall Safety Rating

☐ Safe ☐ Caution ☐ High Risk

Notes

DAILY SAFETY CHECK **Date: ________________** **Day : ____ of 90**

- Any freezing today? ☐ Yes ☐ No
- Any falls today? ☐ Yes ☐ No

Risk Factors Observed

☐ Fatigue
☐ Medication wearing off
☐ Environmental hazards

Overall Safety Rating

☐ Safe ☐ Caution ☐ High Risk

Notes

.**DAILY SAFETY CHECK** **Date:** ______________ **Day :** ____ **of 90**

- Any freezing today? ☐ Yes ☐ No
- Any falls today? ☐ Yes ☐ No

Risk Factors Observed

☐ Fatigue
☐ Medication wearing off
☐ Environmental hazards

Overall Safety Rating

☐ Safe ☐ Caution ☐ High Risk

Notes

DAILY SAFETY CHECK **Date:** ______________ **Day :** ____ **of 90**

- Any freezing today? ☐ Yes ☐ No
- Any falls today? ☐ Yes ☐ No

Risk Factors Observed

☐ Fatigue
☐ Medication wearing off
☐ Environmental hazards

Overall Safety Rating

☐ Safe ☐ Caution ☐ High Risk

Notes

.DAILY SAFETY CHECK Date: ________________ Day : ____ of 90

- Any freezing today? ☐ Yes ☐ No
- Any falls today? ☐ Yes ☐ No

Risk Factors Observed

☐ Fatigue
☐ Medication wearing off
☐ Environmental hazards

Overall Safety Rating

☐ Safe ☐ Caution ☐ High Risk

Notes

DAILY SAFETY CHECK Date: ________________ Day : ____ of 90

- Any freezing today? ☐ Yes ☐ No
- Any falls today? ☐ Yes ☐ No

Risk Factors Observed

☐ Fatigue
☐ Medication wearing off
☐ Environmental hazards

Overall Safety Rating

☐ Safe ☐ Caution ☐ High Risk

Notes

.DAILY SAFETY CHECK Date: ________________ Day : ____ of 90

- Any freezing today? ☐ Yes ☐ No
- Any falls today? ☐ Yes ☐ No

Risk Factors Observed

☐ Fatigue
☐ Medication wearing off
☐ Environmental hazards

Overall Safety Rating

☐ Safe ☐ Caution ☐ High Risk

Notes

DAILY SAFETY CHECK Date: ________________ Day : ____ of 90

- Any freezing today? ☐ Yes ☐ No
- Any falls today? ☐ Yes ☐ No

Risk Factors Observed

☐ Fatigue
☐ Medication wearing off
☐ Environmental hazards

Overall Safety Rating

☐ Safe ☐ Caution ☐ High Risk

Notes

.DAILY SAFETY CHECK Date: ________________ Day : ____ of 90

- Any freezing today? ☐ Yes ☐ No
- Any falls today? ☐ Yes ☐ No

Risk Factors Observed

☐ Fatigue
☐ Medication wearing off
☐ Environmental hazards

Overall Safety Rating

☐ Safe ☐ Caution ☐ High Risk

Notes

DAILY SAFETY CHECK Date: ________________ Day : ____ of 90

- Any freezing today? ☐ Yes ☐ No
- Any falls today? ☐ Yes ☐ No

Risk Factors Observed

☐ Fatigue
☐ Medication wearing off
☐ Environmental hazards

Overall Safety Rating

☐ Safe ☐ Caution ☐ High Risk

Notes

.DAILY SAFETY CHECK **Date: _______________** **Day : ____ of 90**

- Any freezing today? ☐ Yes ☐ No
- Any falls today? ☐ Yes ☐ No

Risk Factors Observed

☐ Fatigue
☐ Medication wearing off
☐ Environmental hazards

Overall Safety Rating

☐ Safe ☐ Caution ☐ High Risk

Notes

DAILY SAFETY CHECK **Date: _______________** **Day : ____ of 90**

- Any freezing today? ☐ Yes ☐ No
- Any falls today? ☐ Yes ☐ No

Risk Factors Observed

☐ Fatigue
☐ Medication wearing off
☐ Environmental hazards

Overall Safety Rating

☐ Safe ☐ Caution ☐ High Risk

Notes

.DAILY SAFETY CHECK **Date: ______________** **Day : ____ of 90**

- Any freezing today? ☐ Yes ☐ No
- Any falls today? ☐ Yes ☐ No

Risk Factors Observed

☐ Fatigue
☐ Medication wearing off
☐ Environmental hazards

Overall Safety Rating

☐ Safe ☐ Caution ☐ High Risk

Notes

DAILY SAFETY CHECK **Date: ______________** **Day : ____ of 90**

- Any freezing today? ☐ Yes ☐ No
- Any falls today? ☐ Yes ☐ No

Risk Factors Observed

☐ Fatigue
☐ Medication wearing off
☐ Environmental hazards

Overall Safety Rating

☐ Safe ☐ Caution ☐ High Risk

Notes

.**DAILY SAFETY CHECK** **Date: ______________** **Day : ____ of 90**

- Any freezing today? ☐ Yes ☐ No
- Any falls today? ☐ Yes ☐ No

Risk Factors Observed

☐ Fatigue
☐ Medication wearing off
☐ Environmental hazards

Overall Safety Rating

☐ Safe ☐ Caution ☐ High Risk

Notes

DAILY SAFETY CHECK **Date: ______________** **Day : ____ of 90**

- Any freezing today? ☐ Yes ☐ No
- Any falls today? ☐ Yes ☐ No

Risk Factors Observed

☐ Fatigue
☐ Medication wearing off
☐ Environmental hazards

Overall Safety Rating

☐ Safe ☐ Caution ☐ High Risk

Notes

.DAILY SAFETY CHECK   Date: ________________   Day : ____ of 90

- Any freezing today?   ☐ Yes   ☐ No
- Any falls today?   ☐ Yes   ☐ No

Risk Factors Observed

☐ Fatigue
☐ Medication wearing off
☐ Environmental hazards

Overall Safety Rating

☐ Safe   ☐ Caution   ☐ High Risk

Notes

DAILY SAFETY CHECK   Date: ________________   Day : ____ of 90

- Any freezing today?   ☐ Yes   ☐ No
- Any falls today?   ☐ Yes   ☐ No

Risk Factors Observed

☐ Fatigue
☐ Medication wearing off
☐ Environmental hazards

Overall Safety Rating

☐ Safe   ☐ Caution   ☐ High Risk

Notes

.DAILY SAFETY CHECK Date: _______________ Day : ____ of 90

- Any freezing today? ☐ Yes ☐ No
- Any falls today? ☐ Yes ☐ No

Risk Factors Observed

☐ Fatigue
☐ Medication wearing off
☐ Environmental hazards

Overall Safety Rating

☐ Safe ☐ Caution ☐ High Risk

Notes

DAILY SAFETY CHECK Date: _______________ Day : ____ of 90

- Any freezing today? ☐ Yes ☐ No
- Any falls today? ☐ Yes ☐ No

Risk Factors Observed

☐ Fatigue
☐ Medication wearing off
☐ Environmental hazards

Overall Safety Rating

☐ Safe ☐ Caution ☐ High Risk

Notes

.DAILY SAFETY CHECK Date: ______________ Day : ____ of 90

- Any freezing today? ☐ Yes ☐ No
- Any falls today? ☐ Yes ☐ No

Risk Factors Observed

☐ Fatigue
☐ Medication wearing off
☐ Environmental hazards

Overall Safety Rating

☐ Safe ☐ Caution ☐ High Risk

Notes

DAILY SAFETY CHECK Date: ______________ Day : ____ of 90

- Any freezing today? ☐ Yes ☐ No
- Any falls today? ☐ Yes ☐ No

Risk Factors Observed

☐ Fatigue
☐ Medication wearing off
☐ Environmental hazards

Overall Safety Rating

☐ Safe ☐ Caution ☐ High Risk

Notes

.**DAILY SAFETY CHECK** **Date: ________________** **Day : ____ of 90**

- Any freezing today? ☐ Yes ☐ No
- Any falls today? ☐ Yes ☐ No

Risk Factors Observed

☐ Fatigue
☐ Medication wearing off
☐ Environmental hazards

Overall Safety Rating

☐ Safe ☐ Caution ☐ High Risk

Notes

DAILY SAFETY CHECK **Date: ________________** **Day : ____ of 90**

- Any freezing today? ☐ Yes ☐ No
- Any falls today? ☐ Yes ☐ No

Risk Factors Observed

☐ Fatigue
☐ Medication wearing off
☐ Environmental hazards

Overall Safety Rating

☐ Safe ☐ Caution ☐ High Risk

Notes

.DAILY SAFETY CHECK Date: ________________ Day : ____ of 90

- Any freezing today? ☐ Yes ☐ No
- Any falls today? ☐ Yes ☐ No

Risk Factors Observed

☐ Fatigue
☐ Medication wearing off
☐ Environmental hazards

Overall Safety Rating

☐ Safe ☐ Caution ☐ High Risk

Notes

DAILY SAFETY CHECK Date: ________________ Day : ____ of 90

- Any freezing today? ☐ Yes ☐ No
- Any falls today? ☐ Yes ☐ No

Risk Factors Observed

☐ Fatigue
☐ Medication wearing off
☐ Environmental hazards

Overall Safety Rating

☐ Safe ☐ Caution ☐ High Risk

Notes

.**DAILY SAFETY CHECK** **Date:** ______________ **Day :** ____ **of 90**

- Any freezing today? ☐ Yes ☐ No
- Any falls today? ☐ Yes ☐ No

Risk Factors Observed

☐ Fatigue
☐ Medication wearing off
☐ Environmental hazards

Overall Safety Rating

☐ Safe ☐ Caution ☐ High Risk

Notes

DAILY SAFETY CHECK **Date:** ______________ **Day :** ____ **of 90**

- Any freezing today? ☐ Yes ☐ No
- Any falls today? ☐ Yes ☐ No

Risk Factors Observed

☐ Fatigue
☐ Medication wearing off
☐ Environmental hazards

Overall Safety Rating

☐ Safe ☐ Caution ☐ High Risk

Notes

.DAILY SAFETY CHECK Date: ________________ Day : ____ of 90

- Any freezing today? ☐ Yes ☐ No
- Any falls today? ☐ Yes ☐ No

Risk Factors Observed

☐ Fatigue
☐ Medication wearing off
☐ Environmental hazards

Overall Safety Rating

☐ Safe ☐ Caution ☐ High Risk

Notes

DAILY SAFETY CHECK Date: ________________ Day : ____ of 90

- Any freezing today? ☐ Yes ☐ No
- Any falls today? ☐ Yes ☐ No

Risk Factors Observed

☐ Fatigue
☐ Medication wearing off
☐ Environmental hazards

Overall Safety Rating

☐ Safe ☐ Caution ☐ High Risk

Notes

.DAILY SAFETY CHECK Date: ______________ Day : ____ of 90

- Any freezing today? ☐ Yes ☐ No
- Any falls today? ☐ Yes ☐ No

Risk Factors Observed

☐ Fatigue
☐ Medication wearing off
☐ Environmental hazards

Overall Safety Rating

☐ Safe ☐ Caution ☐ High Risk

Notes

DAILY SAFETY CHECK Date: ______________ Day : ____ of 90

- Any freezing today? ☐ Yes ☐ No
- Any falls today? ☐ Yes ☐ No

Risk Factors Observed

☐ Fatigue
☐ Medication wearing off
☐ Environmental hazards

Overall Safety Rating

☐ Safe ☐ Caution ☐ High Risk

Notes

.DAILY SAFETY CHECK Date: _______________ Day : ____ of 90

- Any freezing today? ☐ Yes ☐ No
- Any falls today? ☐ Yes ☐ No

Risk Factors Observed

☐ Fatigue
☐ Medication wearing off
☐ Environmental hazards

Overall Safety Rating

☐ Safe ☐ Caution ☐ High Risk

Notes

DAILY SAFETY CHECK Date: _______________ Day : ____ of 90

- Any freezing today? ☐ Yes ☐ No
- Any falls today? ☐ Yes ☐ No

Risk Factors Observed

☐ Fatigue
☐ Medication wearing off
☐ Environmental hazards

Overall Safety Rating

☐ Safe ☐ Caution ☐ High Risk

Notes

.DAILY SAFETY CHECK   Date: ______________   Day : ____ of 90

- Any freezing today?   ☐ Yes   ☐ No
- Any falls today?   ☐ Yes   ☐ No

Risk Factors Observed

☐ Fatigue
☐ Medication wearing off
☐ Environmental hazards

Overall Safety Rating

☐ Safe   ☐ Caution   ☐ High Risk

Notes

DAILY SAFETY CHECK   Date: ______________   Day : ____ of 90

- Any freezing today?   ☐ Yes   ☐ No
- Any falls today?   ☐ Yes   ☐ No

Risk Factors Observed

☐ Fatigue
☐ Medication wearing off
☐ Environmental hazards

Overall Safety Rating

☐ Safe   ☐ Caution   ☐ High Risk

Notes

.DAILY SAFETY CHECK Date: _______________ Day : ____ of 90

- Any freezing today? ☐ Yes ☐ No
- Any falls today? ☐ Yes ☐ No

Risk Factors Observed

☐ Fatigue
☐ Medication wearing off
☐ Environmental hazards

Overall Safety Rating

☐ Safe ☐ Caution ☐ High Risk

Notes

DAILY SAFETY CHECK Date: _______________ Day : ____ of 90

- Any freezing today? ☐ Yes ☐ No
- Any falls today? ☐ Yes ☐ No

Risk Factors Observed

☐ Fatigue
☐ Medication wearing off
☐ Environmental hazards

Overall Safety Rating

☐ Safe ☐ Caution ☐ High Risk

Notes

.DAILY SAFETY CHECK Date: ________________ Day : ____ of 90

- Any freezing today? ☐ Yes ☐ No
- Any falls today? ☐ Yes ☐ No

Risk Factors Observed

☐ Fatigue
☐ Medication wearing off
☐ Environmental hazards

Overall Safety Rating

☐ Safe ☐ Caution ☐ High Risk

Notes

DAILY SAFETY CHECK Date: ________________ Day : ____ of 90

- Any freezing today? ☐ Yes ☐ No
- Any falls today? ☐ Yes ☐ No

Risk Factors Observed

☐ Fatigue
☐ Medication wearing off
☐ Environmental hazards

Overall Safety Rating

☐ Safe ☐ Caution ☐ High Risk

Notes

.**DAILY SAFETY CHECK** **Date:** ________________ **Day :** ____ **of 90**

- Any freezing today? ☐ Yes ☐ No
- Any falls today? ☐ Yes ☐ No

Risk Factors Observed

☐ Fatigue
☐ Medication wearing off
☐ Environmental hazards

Overall Safety Rating

☐ Safe ☐ Caution ☐ High Risk

Notes

DAILY SAFETY CHECK **Date:** ________________ **Day :** ____ **of 90**

- Any freezing today? ☐ Yes ☐ No
- Any falls today? ☐ Yes ☐ No

Risk Factors Observed

☐ Fatigue
☐ Medication wearing off
☐ Environmental hazards

Overall Safety Rating

☐ Safe ☐ Caution ☐ High Risk

Notes

.DAILY SAFETY CHECK **Date: ______________** **Day : ____ of 90**

- Any freezing today? ☐ Yes ☐ No
- Any falls today? ☐ Yes ☐ No

Risk Factors Observed

☐ Fatigue
☐ Medication wearing off
☐ Environmental hazards

Overall Safety Rating

☐ Safe ☐ Caution ☐ High Risk

Notes

DAILY SAFETY CHECK **Date: ______________** **Day : ____ of 90**

- Any freezing today? ☐ Yes ☐ No
- Any falls today? ☐ Yes ☐ No

Risk Factors Observed

☐ Fatigue
☐ Medication wearing off
☐ Environmental hazards

Overall Safety Rating

☐ Safe ☐ Caution ☐ High Risk

Notes

.DAILY SAFETY CHECK Date: _______________ Day : ____ of 90

- Any freezing today? ☐ Yes ☐ No
- Any falls today? ☐ Yes ☐ No

Risk Factors Observed

☐ Fatigue
☐ Medication wearing off
☐ Environmental hazards

Overall Safety Rating

☐ Safe ☐ Caution ☐ High Risk

Notes

DAILY SAFETY CHECK Date: _______________ Day : ____ of 90

- Any freezing today? ☐ Yes ☐ No
- Any falls today? ☐ Yes ☐ No

Risk Factors Observed

☐ Fatigue
☐ Medication wearing off
☐ Environmental hazards

Overall Safety Rating

☐ Safe ☐ Caution ☐ High Risk

Notes

.**DAILY SAFETY CHECK** **Date:** ________________ **Day :** ____ **of 90**

- Any freezing today? ☐ Yes ☐ No
- Any falls today? ☐ Yes ☐ No

Risk Factors Observed

☐ Fatigue
☐ Medication wearing off
☐ Environmental hazards

Overall Safety Rating

☐ Safe ☐ Caution ☐ High Risk

Notes

DAILY SAFETY CHECK **Date:** ________________ **Day :** ____ **of 90**

- Any freezing today? ☐ Yes ☐ No
- Any falls today? ☐ Yes ☐ No

Risk Factors Observed

☐ Fatigue
☐ Medication wearing off
☐ Environmental hazards

Overall Safety Rating

☐ Safe ☐ Caution ☐ High Risk

Notes

.**DAILY SAFETY CHECK** **Date:** ________________ **Day :** ____ **of 90**

- Any freezing today? ☐ Yes ☐ No
- Any falls today? ☐ Yes ☐ No

Risk Factors Observed

☐ Fatigue
☐ Medication wearing off
☐ Environmental hazards

Overall Safety Rating

☐ Safe ☐ Caution ☐ High Risk

Notes

DAILY SAFETY CHECK **Date:** ________________ **Day :** ____ **of 90**

- Any freezing today? ☐ Yes ☐ No
- Any falls today? ☐ Yes ☐ No

Risk Factors Observed

☐ Fatigue
☐ Medication wearing off
☐ Environmental hazards

Overall Safety Rating

☐ Safe ☐ Caution ☐ High Risk

Notes

.**DAILY SAFETY CHECK** **Date:** ________________ **Day :** ____ **of 90**

- Any freezing today? ☐ Yes ☐ No
- Any falls today? ☐ Yes ☐ No

Risk Factors Observed

☐ Fatigue
☐ Medication wearing off
☐ Environmental hazards

Overall Safety Rating

☐ Safe ☐ Caution ☐ High Risk

Notes

DAILY SAFETY CHECK **Date:** ________________ **Day :** ____ **of 90**

- Any freezing today? ☐ Yes ☐ No
- Any falls today? ☐ Yes ☐ No

Risk Factors Observed

☐ Fatigue
☐ Medication wearing off
☐ Environmental hazards

Overall Safety Rating

☐ Safe ☐ Caution ☐ High Risk

Notes

.DAILY SAFETY CHECK Date: ________________ Day : ____ of 90

- Any freezing today? ☐ Yes ☐ No
- Any falls today? ☐ Yes ☐ No

Risk Factors Observed

☐ Fatigue
☐ Medication wearing off
☐ Environmental hazards

Overall Safety Rating

☐ Safe ☐ Caution ☐ High Risk

Notes

DAILY SAFETY CHECK Date: ________________ Day : ____ of 90

- Any freezing today? ☐ Yes ☐ No
- Any falls today? ☐ Yes ☐ No

Risk Factors Observed

☐ Fatigue
☐ Medication wearing off
☐ Environmental hazards

Overall Safety Rating

☐ Safe ☐ Caution ☐ High Risk

Notes

.**DAILY SAFETY CHECK** **Date:** ________________ **Day : ____ of 90**

- Any freezing today? ☐ Yes ☐ No
- Any falls today? ☐ Yes ☐ No

Risk Factors Observed

☐ Fatigue
☐ Medication wearing off
☐ Environmental hazards

Overall Safety Rating

☐ Safe ☐ Caution ☐ High Risk

Notes

DAILY SAFETY CHECK **Date:** ________________ **Day : ____ of 90**

- Any freezing today? ☐ Yes ☐ No
- Any falls today? ☐ Yes ☐ No

Risk Factors Observed

☐ Fatigue
☐ Medication wearing off
☐ Environmental hazards

Overall Safety Rating

☐ Safe ☐ Caution ☐ High Risk

Notes

.DAILY SAFETY CHECK Date: ______________ Day : ____ of 90

- Any freezing today? ☐ Yes ☐ No
- Any falls today? ☐ Yes ☐ No

Risk Factors Observed

☐ Fatigue
☐ Medication wearing off
☐ Environmental hazards

Overall Safety Rating

☐ Safe ☐ Caution ☐ High Risk

Notes

DAILY SAFETY CHECK Date: ______________ Day : ____ of 90

- Any freezing today? ☐ Yes ☐ No
- Any falls today? ☐ Yes ☐ No

Risk Factors Observed

☐ Fatigue
☐ Medication wearing off
☐ Environmental hazards

Overall Safety Rating

☐ Safe ☐ Caution ☐ High Risk

Notes

.**DAILY SAFETY CHECK** **Date:** ______________ **Day :** ____ **of 90**

- Any freezing today? ☐ Yes ☐ No
- Any falls today? ☐ Yes ☐ No

Risk Factors Observed

☐ Fatigue
☐ Medication wearing off
☐ Environmental hazards

Overall Safety Rating

☐ Safe ☐ Caution ☐ High Risk

Notes

DAILY SAFETY CHECK **Date:** ______________ **Day :** ____ **of 90**

- Any freezing today? ☐ Yes ☐ No
- Any falls today? ☐ Yes ☐ No

Risk Factors Observed

☐ Fatigue
☐ Medication wearing off
☐ Environmental hazards

Overall Safety Rating

☐ Safe ☐ Caution ☐ High Risk

Notes

.DAILY SAFETY CHECK Date: ______________ Day : ____ of 90

- Any freezing today? ☐ Yes ☐ No
- Any falls today? ☐ Yes ☐ No

Risk Factors Observed

☐ Fatigue
☐ Medication wearing off
☐ Environmental hazards

Overall Safety Rating

☐ Safe ☐ Caution ☐ High Risk

Notes

DAILY SAFETY CHECK Date: ______________ Day : ____ of 90

- Any freezing today? ☐ Yes ☐ No
- Any falls today? ☐ Yes ☐ No

Risk Factors Observed

☐ Fatigue
☐ Medication wearing off
☐ Environmental hazards

Overall Safety Rating

☐ Safe ☐ Caution ☐ High Risk

Notes

.DAILY SAFETY CHECK Date: ________________ Day : ____ of 90

- Any freezing today? ☐ Yes ☐ No
- Any falls today? ☐ Yes ☐ No

Risk Factors Observed

☐ Fatigue
☐ Medication wearing off
☐ Environmental hazards

Overall Safety Rating

☐ Safe ☐ Caution ☐ High Risk

Notes

DAILY SAFETY CHECK Date: ________________ Day : ____ of 90

- Any freezing today? ☐ Yes ☐ No
- Any falls today? ☐ Yes ☐ No

Risk Factors Observed

☐ Fatigue
☐ Medication wearing off
☐ Environmental hazards

Overall Safety Rating

☐ Safe ☐ Caution ☐ High Risk

Notes

.DAILY SAFETY CHECK Date: ________________ Day : ____ of 90

- Any freezing today? ☐ Yes ☐ No
- Any falls today? ☐ Yes ☐ No

Risk Factors Observed

☐ Fatigue
☐ Medication wearing off
☐ Environmental hazards

Overall Safety Rating

☐ Safe ☐ Caution ☐ High Risk

Notes

DAILY SAFETY CHECK Date: ________________ Day : ____ of 90

- Any freezing today? ☐ Yes ☐ No
- Any falls today? ☐ Yes ☐ No

Risk Factors Observed

☐ Fatigue
☐ Medication wearing off
☐ Environmental hazards

Overall Safety Rating

☐ Safe ☐ Caution ☐ High Risk

Notes

.DAILY SAFETY CHECK Date: ______________ Day : ____ of 90

- Any freezing today? ☐ Yes ☐ No
- Any falls today? ☐ Yes ☐ No

Risk Factors Observed

☐ Fatigue
☐ Medication wearing off
☐ Environmental hazards

Overall Safety Rating

☐ Safe ☐ Caution ☐ High Risk

Notes

DAILY SAFETY CHECK Date: ______________ Day : ____ of 90

- Any freezing today? ☐ Yes ☐ No
- Any falls today? ☐ Yes ☐ No

Risk Factors Observed

☐ Fatigue
☐ Medication wearing off
☐ Environmental hazards

Overall Safety Rating

☐ Safe ☐ Caution ☐ High Risk

Notes

Section 5 - Weekly Safety Summary & Pattern Insights

(Complete After Every 7 Days)

Purpose of This Section

Daily tracking captures events—but **weekly review reveals patterns**.

Use this page to:

- Identify **triggers and high-risk situations**
- Monitor **changes in fall and freezing frequency**
- Improve **safety planning and prevention**
- Prepare for **doctor discussions**

WEEK DETAILS

Week #: ____________ **Date Range:** _____________ to ______________

INCIDENT OVERVIEW

Total Falls: ________ Total Near-Falls: ________ Total Freezing Episodes: ______

SAFETY TREND

Compared to last week:

☐ Improving ☐ Stable ☐ Worsening

KEY TRIGGERS IDENTIFIED

☐ Turning ☐ Doorways / narrow spaces ☐ Fatigue
☐ Medication wearing off ☐ Clutter or obstacles ☐ Poor lighting
☐ Stress or distraction Other: ____

HIGH-RISK TIMES

Most incidents occurred at: ☐ Morning ☐ Afternoon ☐ Evening ☐ Night

Specific time (if known): _________________________

FREEZING PATTERN INSIGHTS

Most common activity during freezing:

Average severity: ☐ Mild ☐ Moderate ☐ Severe

Change from last week: ☐ Improved ☐ Same ☐ Worsened

FALL ANALYSIS

Most common cause: ____

Were injuries involved? ☐ Yes ☐ No

Details: ____

MEDICATION OBSERVATIONS

- Medication taken on time: ☐ Always ☐ Mostly ☐ Sometimes ☐ Rarely
- Wearing-off periods noticed: ☐ Yes ☐ No
- Link between medication timing and incidents: ___________________________

EARLY WARNING SIGNS OBSERVED

☐ Increased freezing ☐ Reduced balance ☐ Slower movement
☐ Increased fatigue ☐ Reduced confidence walking

CAREGIVER NOTES

What stood out this week?

____

____

CAREGIVER CHECK-IN

- Stress Level (1–10): ________
- Energy Level (1–10): ________

What helped you most this week?

____

ACTION PLAN FOR NEXT WEEK

☐ Improve lighting / environment
☐ Remove hazards
☐ Adjust daily routine
☐ Monitor high-risk times
☐ Review medication timing

Other: ____

QUESTIONS FOR DOCTOR

____

____

____

WEEKLY REFLECTION

Small patterns can lead to big improvements.
Consistent tracking helps create a safer environment over time.

____

WEEK DETAILS

Week #: ____________ **Date Range:** _____________ to ______________

INCIDENT OVERVIEW

Total Falls: ________ Total Near-Falls: ________ Total Freezing Episodes: ______

SAFETY TREND

Compared to last week:

☐ Improving ☐ Stable ☐ Worsening

KEY TRIGGERS IDENTIFIED

☐ Turning ☐ Doorways / narrow spaces ☐ Fatigue
☐ Medication wearing off ☐ Clutter or obstacles ☐ Poor lighting
☐ Stress or distraction Other: ____

HIGH-RISK TIMES

Most incidents occurred at: ☐ Morning ☐ Afternoon ☐ Evening ☐ Night

Specific time (if known): _________________________

FREEZING PATTERN INSIGHTS

Most common activity during freezing:

Average severity: ☐ Mild ☐ Moderate ☐ Severe

Change from last week: ☐ Improved ☐ Same ☐ Worsened

FALL ANALYSIS

Most common cause: ____

Were injuries involved? ☐ Yes ☐ No

Details: ____

MEDICATION OBSERVATIONS

- Medication taken on time: ☐ Always ☐ Mostly ☐ Sometimes ☐ Rarely
- Wearing-off periods noticed: ☐ Yes ☐ No
- Link between medication timing and incidents: __________________________

EARLY WARNING SIGNS OBSERVED

☐ Increased freezing ☐ Reduced balance ☐ Slower movement
☐ Increased fatigue ☐ Reduced confidence walking

CAREGIVER NOTES

What stood out this week?

____

____

CAREGIVER CHECK-IN

- Stress Level (1–10): ________
- Energy Level (1–10): ________

What helped you most this week?

____

ACTION PLAN FOR NEXT WEEK

☐ Improve lighting / environment
☐ Remove hazards
☐ Adjust daily routine
☐ Monitor high-risk times
☐ Review medication timing

Other: ____

QUESTIONS FOR DOCTOR

____

____

____

WEEKLY REFLECTION

Small patterns can lead to big improvements.
Consistent tracking helps create a safer environment over time.

____

WEEK DETAILS

Week #: ____________ **Date Range:** _____________ to ______________

INCIDENT OVERVIEW

Total Falls: ________ Total Near-Falls: ________ Total Freezing Episodes: ______

SAFETY TREND

Compared to last week:

☐ Improving ☐ Stable ☐ Worsening

KEY TRIGGERS IDENTIFIED

☐ Turning ☐ Doorways / narrow spaces ☐ Fatigue
☐ Medication wearing off ☐ Clutter or obstacles ☐ Poor lighting
☐ Stress or distraction Other: ____

HIGH-RISK TIMES

Most incidents occurred at: ☐ Morning ☐ Afternoon ☐ Evening ☐ Night

Specific time (if known): _________________________

FREEZING PATTERN INSIGHTS

Most common activity during freezing:

Average severity: ☐ Mild ☐ Moderate ☐ Severe

Change from last week: ☐ Improved ☐ Same ☐ Worsened

FALL ANALYSIS

Most common cause: ____

Were injuries involved? ☐ Yes ☐ No

Details: ____

MEDICATION OBSERVATIONS

- Medication taken on time: ☐ Always ☐ Mostly ☐ Sometimes ☐ Rarely
- Wearing-off periods noticed: ☐ Yes ☐ No
- Link between medication timing and incidents: ___________________________

EARLY WARNING SIGNS OBSERVED

☐ Increased freezing ☐ Reduced balance ☐ Slower movement
☐ Increased fatigue ☐ Reduced confidence walking

CAREGIVER NOTES

What stood out this week?

CAREGIVER CHECK-IN

- Stress Level (1–10): ________
- Energy Level (1–10): ________

What helped you most this week?

ACTION PLAN FOR NEXT WEEK

☐ Improve lighting / environment
☐ Remove hazards
☐ Adjust daily routine
☐ Monitor high-risk times
☐ Review medication timing

Other: ____

QUESTIONS FOR DOCTOR

WEEKLY REFLECTION

Small patterns can lead to big improvements.
Consistent tracking helps create a safer environment over time.

WEEK DETAILS

Week #: ____________ **Date Range:** ____________ to ______________

INCIDENT OVERVIEW

Total Falls: ________ Total Near-Falls: ________ Total Freezing Episodes: ______

SAFETY TREND

Compared to last week:

☐ Improving ☐ Stable ☐ Worsening

KEY TRIGGERS IDENTIFIED

☐ Turning ☐ Doorways / narrow spaces ☐ Fatigue
☐ Medication wearing off ☐ Clutter or obstacles ☐ Poor lighting
☐ Stress or distraction Other: ____

HIGH-RISK TIMES

Most incidents occurred at: ☐ Morning ☐ Afternoon ☐ Evening ☐ Night

Specific time (if known): _________________________

FREEZING PATTERN INSIGHTS

Most common activity during freezing:

Average severity: ☐ Mild ☐ Moderate ☐ Severe

Change from last week: ☐ Improved ☐ Same ☐ Worsened

FALL ANALYSIS

Most common cause: ____

Were injuries involved? ☐ Yes ☐ No

Details: ____

MEDICATION OBSERVATIONS

- Medication taken on time: ☐ Always ☐ Mostly ☐ Sometimes ☐ Rarely
- Wearing-off periods noticed: ☐ Yes ☐ No
- Link between medication timing and incidents: ___________________________

EARLY WARNING SIGNS OBSERVED

☐ Increased freezing ☐ Reduced balance ☐ Slower movement
☐ Increased fatigue ☐ Reduced confidence walking

CAREGIVER NOTES

What stood out this week?

CAREGIVER CHECK-IN

- Stress Level (1–10): ________
- Energy Level (1–10): ________

What helped you most this week?

ACTION PLAN FOR NEXT WEEK

☐ Improve lighting / environment
☐ Remove hazards
☐ Adjust daily routine
☐ Monitor high-risk times
☐ Review medication timing

Other: ____

QUESTIONS FOR DOCTOR

WEEKLY REFLECTION

Small patterns can lead to big improvements.
Consistent tracking helps create a safer environment over time.

WEEK DETAILS

Week #: ____________ **Date Range:** _____________ to ______________

INCIDENT OVERVIEW

Total Falls: ________ Total Near-Falls: ________ Total Freezing Episodes: ______

SAFETY TREND

Compared to last week:

☐ Improving ☐ Stable ☐ Worsening

KEY TRIGGERS IDENTIFIED

☐ Turning ☐ Doorways / narrow spaces ☐ Fatigue
☐ Medication wearing off ☐ Clutter or obstacles ☐ Poor lighting
☐ Stress or distraction Other: ____

HIGH-RISK TIMES

Most incidents occurred at: ☐ Morning ☐ Afternoon ☐ Evening ☐ Night

Specific time (if known): _________________________

FREEZING PATTERN INSIGHTS

Most common activity during freezing:

Average severity: ☐ Mild ☐ Moderate ☐ Severe

Change from last week: ☐ Improved ☐ Same ☐ Worsened

FALL ANALYSIS

Most common cause: ____

Were injuries involved? ☐ Yes ☐ No

Details: ____

MEDICATION OBSERVATIONS

- Medication taken on time: ☐ Always ☐ Mostly ☐ Sometimes ☐ Rarely
- Wearing-off periods noticed: ☐ Yes ☐ No
- Link between medication timing and incidents: ___________________________

EARLY WARNING SIGNS OBSERVED

☐ Increased freezing ☐ Reduced balance ☐ Slower movement

☐ Increased fatigue ☐ Reduced confidence walking

CAREGIVER NOTES

What stood out this week?

____

____

CAREGIVER CHECK-IN

- Stress Level (1–10): ________
- Energy Level (1–10): ________

What helped you most this week?

____

ACTION PLAN FOR NEXT WEEK

☐ Improve lighting / environment
☐ Remove hazards
☐ Adjust daily routine
☐ Monitor high-risk times
☐ Review medication timing

Other: ____

QUESTIONS FOR DOCTOR

____

____

____

WEEKLY REFLECTION

Small patterns can lead to big improvements.
Consistent tracking helps create a safer environment over time.

____

WEEK DETAILS

Week #: ____________ **Date Range:** _____________ to ______________

INCIDENT OVERVIEW

Total Falls: ________ Total Near-Falls: ________ Total Freezing Episodes: ______

SAFETY TREND

Compared to last week:

☐ Improving ☐ Stable ☐ Worsening

KEY TRIGGERS IDENTIFIED

☐ Turning ☐ Doorways / narrow spaces ☐ Fatigue
☐ Medication wearing off ☐ Clutter or obstacles ☐ Poor lighting
☐ Stress or distraction Other: ____

HIGH-RISK TIMES

Most incidents occurred at: ☐ Morning ☐ Afternoon ☐ Evening ☐ Night

Specific time (if known): _________________________

FREEZING PATTERN INSIGHTS

Most common activity during freezing:

Average severity: ☐ Mild ☐ Moderate ☐ Severe

Change from last week: ☐ Improved ☐ Same ☐ Worsened

FALL ANALYSIS

Most common cause: ____

Were injuries involved? ☐ Yes ☐ No

Details: ____

MEDICATION OBSERVATIONS

- Medication taken on time: ☐ Always ☐ Mostly ☐ Sometimes ☐ Rarely
- Wearing-off periods noticed: ☐ Yes ☐ No
- Link between medication timing and incidents: __________________________

EARLY WARNING SIGNS OBSERVED

☐ Increased freezing ☐ Reduced balance ☐ Slower movement
☐ Increased fatigue ☐ Reduced confidence walking

CAREGIVER NOTES

What stood out this week?

CAREGIVER CHECK-IN

- Stress Level (1–10): ________
- Energy Level (1–10): ________

What helped you most this week?

ACTION PLAN FOR NEXT WEEK

☐ Improve lighting / environment
☐ Remove hazards
☐ Adjust daily routine
☐ Monitor high-risk times
☐ Review medication timing

Other: ____

QUESTIONS FOR DOCTOR

WEEKLY REFLECTION

Small patterns can lead to big improvements.
Consistent tracking helps create a safer environment over time.

WEEK DETAILS

Week #: ____________ **Date Range:** ____________ to ______________

INCIDENT OVERVIEW

Total Falls: ________ Total Near-Falls: ________ Total Freezing Episodes: ______

SAFETY TREND

Compared to last week:

☐ Improving ☐ Stable ☐ Worsening

KEY TRIGGERS IDENTIFIED

☐ Turning ☐ Doorways / narrow spaces ☐ Fatigue
☐ Medication wearing off ☐ Clutter or obstacles ☐ Poor lighting
☐ Stress or distraction Other: ____

HIGH-RISK TIMES

Most incidents occurred at: ☐ Morning ☐ Afternoon ☐ Evening ☐ Night

Specific time (if known): _________________________

FREEZING PATTERN INSIGHTS

Most common activity during freezing:

Average severity: ☐ Mild ☐ Moderate ☐ Severe

Change from last week: ☐ Improved ☐ Same ☐ Worsened

FALL ANALYSIS

Most common cause: ____

Were injuries involved? ☐ Yes ☐ No

Details: ____

MEDICATION OBSERVATIONS

- Medication taken on time: ☐ Always ☐ Mostly ☐ Sometimes ☐ Rarely
- Wearing-off periods noticed: ☐ Yes ☐ No
- Link between medication timing and incidents: ___________________________

EARLY WARNING SIGNS OBSERVED

☐ Increased freezing ☐ Reduced balance ☐ Slower movement
☐ Increased fatigue ☐ Reduced confidence walking

CAREGIVER NOTES

What stood out this week?

____

____

CAREGIVER CHECK-IN

- Stress Level (1–10): ________
- Energy Level (1–10): ________

What helped you most this week?

____

ACTION PLAN FOR NEXT WEEK

☐ Improve lighting / environment
☐ Remove hazards
☐ Adjust daily routine
☐ Monitor high-risk times
☐ Review medication timing

Other: ______________________________

QUESTIONS FOR DOCTOR

____

____

____

WEEKLY REFLECTION

Small patterns can lead to big improvements.
Consistent tracking helps create a safer environment over time.

____

WEEK DETAILS

Week #: ____________ **Date Range:** _____________ to ______________

INCIDENT OVERVIEW

Total Falls: ________ Total Near-Falls: ________ Total Freezing Episodes: ______

SAFETY TREND

Compared to last week:

☐ Improving ☐ Stable ☐ Worsening

KEY TRIGGERS IDENTIFIED

☐ Turning ☐ Doorways / narrow spaces ☐ Fatigue
☐ Medication wearing off ☐ Clutter or obstacles ☐ Poor lighting
☐ Stress or distraction Other: ____

HIGH-RISK TIMES

Most incidents occurred at: ☐ Morning ☐ Afternoon ☐ Evening ☐ Night

Specific time (if known): _________________________

FREEZING PATTERN INSIGHTS

Most common activity during freezing:

Average severity: ☐ Mild ☐ Moderate ☐ Severe

Change from last week: ☐ Improved ☐ Same ☐ Worsened

FALL ANALYSIS

Most common cause: ____

Were injuries involved? ☐ Yes ☐ No

Details: ____

MEDICATION OBSERVATIONS

- Medication taken on time: ☐ Always ☐ Mostly ☐ Sometimes ☐ Rarely
- Wearing-off periods noticed: ☐ Yes ☐ No
- Link between medication timing and incidents: ___________________________

EARLY WARNING SIGNS OBSERVED

☐ Increased freezing ☐ Reduced balance ☐ Slower movement
☐ Increased fatigue ☐ Reduced confidence walking

CAREGIVER NOTES

What stood out this week?

____

____

CAREGIVER CHECK-IN

- Stress Level (1–10): ________
- Energy Level (1–10): ________

What helped you most this week?

____

ACTION PLAN FOR NEXT WEEK

☐ Improve lighting / environment
☐ Remove hazards
☐ Adjust daily routine
☐ Monitor high-risk times
☐ Review medication timing

Other: ______________________________

QUESTIONS FOR DOCTOR

____

____

____

WEEKLY REFLECTION

Small patterns can lead to big improvements.
Consistent tracking helps create a safer environment over time.

____

WEEK DETAILS

Week #: ____________ **Date Range:** _____________ to ______________

INCIDENT OVERVIEW

Total Falls: ________ Total Near-Falls: ________ Total Freezing Episodes: ______

SAFETY TREND

Compared to last week:

☐ Improving ☐ Stable ☐ Worsening

KEY TRIGGERS IDENTIFIED

☐ Turning ☐ Doorways / narrow spaces ☐ Fatigue
☐ Medication wearing off ☐ Clutter or obstacles ☐ Poor lighting
☐ Stress or distraction Other: ____

HIGH-RISK TIMES

Most incidents occurred at: ☐ Morning ☐ Afternoon ☐ Evening ☐ Night

Specific time (if known): _________________________

FREEZING PATTERN INSIGHTS

Most common activity during freezing:

Average severity: ☐ Mild ☐ Moderate ☐ Severe

Change from last week: ☐ Improved ☐ Same ☐ Worsened

FALL ANALYSIS

Most common cause: ____

Were injuries involved? ☐ Yes ☐ No

Details: ____

MEDICATION OBSERVATIONS

- Medication taken on time: ☐ Always ☐ Mostly ☐ Sometimes ☐ Rarely
- Wearing-off periods noticed: ☐ Yes ☐ No
- Link between medication timing and incidents: ___________________________

EARLY WARNING SIGNS OBSERVED

☐ Increased freezing ☐ Reduced balance ☐ Slower movement
☐ Increased fatigue ☐ Reduced confidence walking

CAREGIVER NOTES

What stood out this week?

CAREGIVER CHECK-IN

- Stress Level (1–10): ________
- Energy Level (1–10): ________

What helped you most this week?

ACTION PLAN FOR NEXT WEEK

☐ Improve lighting / environment
☐ Remove hazards
☐ Adjust daily routine
☐ Monitor high-risk times
☐ Review medication timing

Other: ____

QUESTIONS FOR DOCTOR

WEEKLY REFLECTION

Small patterns can lead to big improvements.
Consistent tracking helps create a safer environment over time.

WEEK DETAILS

Week #: ____________ **Date Range:** ____________ to ______________

INCIDENT OVERVIEW

Total Falls: _________ Total Near-Falls: ________ Total Freezing Episodes: ______

SAFETY TREND

Compared to last week:

☐ Improving ☐ Stable ☐ Worsening

KEY TRIGGERS IDENTIFIED

☐ Turning ☐ Doorways / narrow spaces ☐ Fatigue
☐ Medication wearing off ☐ Clutter or obstacles ☐ Poor lighting
☐ Stress or distraction Other: ____

HIGH-RISK TIMES

Most incidents occurred at: ☐ Morning ☐ Afternoon ☐ Evening ☐ Night

Specific time (if known): ________________________

FREEZING PATTERN INSIGHTS

Most common activity during freezing:

Average severity: ☐ Mild ☐ Moderate ☐ Severe

Change from last week: ☐ Improved ☐ Same ☐ Worsened

FALL ANALYSIS

Most common cause: ____

Were injuries involved? ☐ Yes ☐ No

Details: ____

MEDICATION OBSERVATIONS

- Medication taken on time: ☐ Always ☐ Mostly ☐ Sometimes ☐ Rarely
- Wearing-off periods noticed: ☐ Yes ☐ No
- Link between medication timing and incidents: __________________________

EARLY WARNING SIGNS OBSERVED

☐ Increased freezing ☐ Reduced balance ☐ Slower movement
☐ Increased fatigue ☐ Reduced confidence walking

CAREGIVER NOTES

What stood out this week?

____

____

CAREGIVER CHECK-IN

- Stress Level (1–10): ________
- Energy Level (1–10): ________

What helped you most this week?

____

ACTION PLAN FOR NEXT WEEK

☐ Improve lighting / environment
☐ Remove hazards
☐ Adjust daily routine
☐ Monitor high-risk times
☐ Review medication timing

Other: ____

QUESTIONS FOR DOCTOR

____

____

____

WEEKLY REFLECTION

Small patterns can lead to big improvements.
Consistent tracking helps create a safer environment over time.

____

WEEK DETAILS

Week #: ____________ **Date Range:** _____________ to ______________

INCIDENT OVERVIEW

Total Falls: ________ Total Near-Falls: ________ Total Freezing Episodes: ______

SAFETY TREND

Compared to last week:

☐ Improving ☐ Stable ☐ Worsening

KEY TRIGGERS IDENTIFIED

☐ Turning ☐ Doorways / narrow spaces ☐ Fatigue
☐ Medication wearing off ☐ Clutter or obstacles ☐ Poor lighting
☐ Stress or distraction Other: ____

HIGH-RISK TIMES

Most incidents occurred at: ☐ Morning ☐ Afternoon ☐ Evening ☐ Night

Specific time (if known): _________________________

FREEZING PATTERN INSIGHTS

Most common activity during freezing:

Average severity: ☐ Mild ☐ Moderate ☐ Severe

Change from last week: ☐ Improved ☐ Same ☐ Worsened

FALL ANALYSIS

Most common cause: ____

Were injuries involved? ☐ Yes ☐ No

Details: ____

MEDICATION OBSERVATIONS

- Medication taken on time: ☐ Always ☐ Mostly ☐ Sometimes ☐ Rarely
- Wearing-off periods noticed: ☐ Yes ☐ No
- Link between medication timing and incidents: ___________________________

EARLY WARNING SIGNS OBSERVED

☐ Increased freezing ☐ Reduced balance ☐ Slower movement
☐ Increased fatigue ☐ Reduced confidence walking

CAREGIVER NOTES

What stood out this week?

____

____

CAREGIVER CHECK-IN

- Stress Level (1–10): ________
- Energy Level (1–10): ________

What helped you most this week?

____

ACTION PLAN FOR NEXT WEEK

☐ Improve lighting / environment
☐ Remove hazards
☐ Adjust daily routine
☐ Monitor high-risk times
☐ Review medication timing

Other: ______________________________

QUESTIONS FOR DOCTOR

____

____

____

WEEKLY REFLECTION

Small patterns can lead to big improvements.
Consistent tracking helps create a safer environment over time.

____

WEEK DETAILS

Week #: ____________ **Date Range:** ____________ to ______________

INCIDENT OVERVIEW

Total Falls: ________ Total Near-Falls: ________ Total Freezing Episodes: ______

SAFETY TREND

Compared to last week:

☐ Improving ☐ Stable ☐ Worsening

KEY TRIGGERS IDENTIFIED

☐ Turning ☐ Doorways / narrow spaces ☐ Fatigue
☐ Medication wearing off ☐ Clutter or obstacles ☐ Poor lighting
☐ Stress or distraction Other: ____________________________________

HIGH-RISK TIMES

Most incidents occurred at: ☐ Morning ☐ Afternoon ☐ Evening ☐ Night

Specific time (if known): _________________________

FREEZING PATTERN INSIGHTS

Most common activity during freezing:

Average severity: ☐ Mild ☐ Moderate ☐ Severe

Change from last week: ☐ Improved ☐ Same ☐ Worsened

FALL ANALYSIS

Most common cause: ____

Were injuries involved? ☐ Yes ☐ No

Details: ____

MEDICATION OBSERVATIONS

- Medication taken on time: ☐ Always ☐ Mostly ☐ Sometimes ☐ Rarely
- Wearing-off periods noticed: ☐ Yes ☐ No
- Link between medication timing and incidents: ___________________________

EARLY WARNING SIGNS OBSERVED

☐ Increased freezing ☐ Reduced balance ☐ Slower movement
☐ Increased fatigue ☐ Reduced confidence walking

CAREGIVER NOTES

What stood out this week?

____

____

CAREGIVER CHECK-IN

- Stress Level (1–10): ________
- Energy Level (1–10): ________

What helped you most this week?

____

ACTION PLAN FOR NEXT WEEK

☐ Improve lighting / environment
☐ Remove hazards
☐ Adjust daily routine
☐ Monitor high-risk times
☐ Review medication timing

Other: ____

QUESTIONS FOR DOCTOR

____

____

____

WEEKLY REFLECTION

Small patterns can lead to big improvements.
Consistent tracking helps create a safer environment over time.

____

Section 10 - Doctor Visits & Medical Notes

(Use this section to prepare for appointments, track medical advice, and ensure nothing important is missed.)

HOW TO USE THIS PAGE

- Prepare key questions before each visit
- Record doctor recommendations and changes
- Track medications, symptoms, and follow-ups
- Bring this page to every appointment

APPOINTMENT DETAILS

Patient Name: ______________________ **Date of Visit:** __________________________
Doctor / Specialist: ___________________ **Clinic / Hospital:** _____________________

Reason for Visit: __________________________

SYMPTOM SUMMARY (TO DISCUSS) *(List key concerns since last visit)*

QUESTIONS FOR THE DOCTOR

1.
2.
3.

DOCTOR'S OBSERVATIONS & DIAGNOSIS

MEDICATION REVIEW

Medication	Change (Start/Stop/Adjust)	Dosage	Notes

TREATMENT PLAN / RECOMMENDATIONS

☐ Physical Therapy ☐ Lifestyle Changes ☐ New Medication
☐ Tests Required ☐ Specialist Referral ☐ Other: _______

Details:

TESTS & RESULTS

Test	Date	Result	Notes

FOLLOW-UP PLAN

Next Appointment Date: ____________________

Things to Monitor Until Next Visit:

Pro Care Insight:
Clear communication with healthcare providers leads to better treatment decisions and improved patient outcomes.

APPOINTMENT DETAILS

Patient Name: ______________________ **Date of Visit:** ________________________
Doctor / Specialist: __________________ **Clinic / Hospital:** ____________________

Reason for Visit: _________________________

SYMPTOM SUMMARY (TO DISCUSS) *(List key concerns since last visit)*

QUESTIONS FOR THE DOCTOR

1. ____
2. ____
3. ____

DOCTOR'S OBSERVATIONS & DIAGNOSIS

MEDICATION REVIEW

Medication	Change (Start/Stop/Adjust)	Dosage	Notes

TREATMENT PLAN / RECOMMENDATIONS

☐ Physical Therapy ☐ Lifestyle Changes ☐ New Medication
☐ Tests Required ☐ Specialist Referral ☐ Other: _______

Details:

TESTS & RESULTS

Test	Date	Result	Notes

FOLLOW-UP PLAN

Next Appointment Date: ____________________

Things to Monitor Until Next Visit:

____

Pro Care Insight:
Clear communication with healthcare providers leads to better treatment decisions and improved patient outcomes.

APPOINTMENT DETAILS

Patient Name: ______________________ **Date of Visit:** ________________________
Doctor / Specialist: __________________ **Clinic / Hospital:** ____________________

Reason for Visit: _________________________

SYMPTOM SUMMARY (TO DISCUSS) *(List key concerns since last visit)*

QUESTIONS FOR THE DOCTOR

1.
2.
3.

DOCTOR'S OBSERVATIONS & DIAGNOSIS

MEDICATION REVIEW

Medication	Change (Start/Stop/Adjust)	Dosage	Notes

TREATMENT PLAN / RECOMMENDATIONS

☐ Physical Therapy ☐ Lifestyle Changes ☐ New Medication
☐ Tests Required ☐ Specialist Referral ☐ Other: _______

Details:

TESTS & RESULTS

Test	Date	Result	Notes

FOLLOW-UP PLAN

Next Appointment Date: ____________________

Things to Monitor Until Next Visit:

Pro Care Insight:
Clear communication with healthcare providers leads to better treatment decisions and improved patient outcomes.

APPOINTMENT DETAILS

Patient Name: ______________________ **Date of Visit:** _________________________
Doctor / Specialist: __________________ **Clinic / Hospital:** _____________________

Reason for Visit: _________________________

SYMPTOM SUMMARY (TO DISCUSS) *(List key concerns since last visit)*

QUESTIONS FOR THE DOCTOR

1. ____
2. ____
3. ____

DOCTOR'S OBSERVATIONS & DIAGNOSIS

MEDICATION REVIEW

Medication	Change (Start/Stop/Adjust)	Dosage	Notes

TREATMENT PLAN / RECOMMENDATIONS

☐ Physical Therapy ☐ Lifestyle Changes ☐ New Medication
☐ Tests Required ☐ Specialist Referral ☐ Other: _______

Details:

TESTS & RESULTS

Test	Date	Result	Notes

FOLLOW-UP PLAN

Next Appointment Date: ____________________

Things to Monitor Until Next Visit:

____

Pro Care Insight:
Clear communication with healthcare providers leads to better treatment decisions and improved patient outcomes.

APPOINTMENT DETAILS

Patient Name: ______________________ **Date of Visit:** ________________________

Doctor / Specialist: __________________ **Clinic / Hospital:** ____________________

Reason for Visit: _________________________

SYMPTOM SUMMARY (TO DISCUSS) *(List key concerns since last visit)*

QUESTIONS FOR THE DOCTOR

1. ____
2. ____
3. ____

DOCTOR'S OBSERVATIONS & DIAGNOSIS

MEDICATION REVIEW

Medication	Change (Start/Stop/Adjust)	Dosage	Notes

TREATMENT PLAN / RECOMMENDATIONS

☐ Physical Therapy ☐ Lifestyle Changes ☐ New Medication

☐ Tests Required ☐ Specialist Referral ☐ Other: _______

Details:

TESTS & RESULTS

Test	Date	Result	Notes

FOLLOW-UP PLAN

Next Appointment Date: ____________________

Things to Monitor Until Next Visit:

____

Pro Care Insight:
Clear communication with healthcare providers leads to better treatment decisions and improved patient outcomes.

APPOINTMENT DETAILS

Patient Name: ______________________ **Date of Visit:** ________________________
Doctor / Specialist: __________________ **Clinic / Hospital:** ____________________

Reason for Visit: _________________________

SYMPTOM SUMMARY (TO DISCUSS) *(List key concerns since last visit)*

QUESTIONS FOR THE DOCTOR

1.
2.
3.

DOCTOR'S OBSERVATIONS & DIAGNOSIS

MEDICATION REVIEW

Medication	Change (Start/Stop/Adjust)	Dosage	Notes

TREATMENT PLAN / RECOMMENDATIONS

☐ Physical Therapy ☐ Lifestyle Changes ☐ New Medication
☐ Tests Required ☐ Specialist Referral ☐ Other: _______

Details:

TESTS & RESULTS

Test	Date	Result	Notes

FOLLOW-UP PLAN

Next Appointment Date: ____________________

Things to Monitor Until Next Visit:

Pro Care Insight:
Clear communication with healthcare providers leads to better treatment decisions and improved patient outcomes.

APPOINTMENT DETAILS

Patient Name: ______________________ **Date of Visit:** ________________________
Doctor / Specialist: __________________ **Clinic / Hospital:** ____________________

Reason for Visit: _________________________

SYMPTOM SUMMARY (TO DISCUSS) *(List key concerns since last visit)*

QUESTIONS FOR THE DOCTOR

1. ____
2. ____
3. ____

DOCTOR'S OBSERVATIONS & DIAGNOSIS

MEDICATION REVIEW

Medication	Change (Start/Stop/Adjust)	Dosage	Notes

TREATMENT PLAN / RECOMMENDATIONS

☐ Physical Therapy ☐ Lifestyle Changes ☐ New Medication
☐ Tests Required ☐ Specialist Referral ☐ Other: _______

Details:

TESTS & RESULTS

Test	Date	Result	Notes

FOLLOW-UP PLAN

Next Appointment Date: ____________________

Things to Monitor Until Next Visit:

____

Pro Care Insight:
Clear communication with healthcare providers leads to better treatment decisions and improved patient outcomes.

APPOINTMENT DETAILS

Patient Name: ______________________ **Date of Visit:** ________________________
Doctor / Specialist: __________________ **Clinic / Hospital:** ____________________

Reason for Visit: _________________________

SYMPTOM SUMMARY (TO DISCUSS) *(List key concerns since last visit)*

QUESTIONS FOR THE DOCTOR

1.
2.
3.

DOCTOR'S OBSERVATIONS & DIAGNOSIS

MEDICATION REVIEW

Medication	Change (Start/Stop/Adjust)	Dosage	Notes

TREATMENT PLAN / RECOMMENDATIONS

☐ Physical Therapy ☐ Lifestyle Changes ☐ New Medication
☐ Tests Required ☐ Specialist Referral ☐ Other: _______

Details:

TESTS & RESULTS

Test	Date	Result	Notes

FOLLOW-UP PLAN

Next Appointment Date: ____________________

Things to Monitor Until Next Visit:

Pro Care Insight:
Clear communication with healthcare providers leads to better treatment decisions and improved patient outcomes.

APPOINTMENT DETAILS

Patient Name: ______________________ **Date of Visit:** ________________________
Doctor / Specialist: __________________ **Clinic / Hospital:** ____________________

Reason for Visit: _________________________

SYMPTOM SUMMARY (TO DISCUSS) *(List key concerns since last visit)*

QUESTIONS FOR THE DOCTOR

1. ______________________________
2. ______________________________
3. ______________________________

DOCTOR'S OBSERVATIONS & DIAGNOSIS

MEDICATION REVIEW

Medication	Change (Start/Stop/Adjust)	Dosage	Notes

TREATMENT PLAN / RECOMMENDATIONS

☐ Physical Therapy ☐ Lifestyle Changes ☐ New Medication
☐ Tests Required ☐ Specialist Referral ☐ Other: _______

Details:

TESTS & RESULTS

Test	Date	Result	Notes

FOLLOW-UP PLAN

Next Appointment Date: ____________________

Things to Monitor Until Next Visit:

____

Pro Care Insight:
Clear communication with healthcare providers leads to better treatment decisions and improved patient outcomes.

APPOINTMENT DETAILS

Patient Name: ______________________ **Date of Visit:** ________________________
Doctor / Specialist: __________________ **Clinic / Hospital:** ____________________

Reason for Visit: _________________________

SYMPTOM SUMMARY (TO DISCUSS) *(List key concerns since last visit)*

QUESTIONS FOR THE DOCTOR

1. ____

2. ____

3. ____

DOCTOR'S OBSERVATIONS & DIAGNOSIS

MEDICATION REVIEW

Medication	Change (Start/Stop/Adjust)	Dosage	Notes

TREATMENT PLAN / RECOMMENDATIONS

☐ Physical Therapy ☐ Lifestyle Changes ☐ New Medication
☐ Tests Required ☐ Specialist Referral ☐ Other: _______

Details:

TESTS & RESULTS

Test	Date	Result	Notes

FOLLOW-UP PLAN

Next Appointment Date: ____________________

Things to Monitor Until Next Visit:

____

Pro Care Insight:
Clear communication with healthcare providers leads to better treatment decisions and improved patient outcomes.

APPOINTMENT DETAILS

Patient Name: ______________________ **Date of Visit:** ________________________
Doctor / Specialist: __________________ **Clinic / Hospital:** ____________________

Reason for Visit: _________________________

SYMPTOM SUMMARY (TO DISCUSS) *(List key concerns since last visit)*

QUESTIONS FOR THE DOCTOR

1. ____
2. ____
3. ____

DOCTOR'S OBSERVATIONS & DIAGNOSIS

MEDICATION REVIEW

Medication	Change (Start/Stop/Adjust)	Dosage	Notes

TREATMENT PLAN / RECOMMENDATIONS

☐ Physical Therapy ☐ Lifestyle Changes ☐ New Medication
☐ Tests Required ☐ Specialist Referral ☐ Other: _______

Details:

TESTS & RESULTS

Test	Date	Result	Notes

FOLLOW-UP PLAN

Next Appointment Date: ____________________

Things to Monitor Until Next Visit:

____

Pro Care Insight:
Clear communication with healthcare providers leads to better treatment decisions and improved patient outcomes.

APPOINTMENT DETAILS

Patient Name: ______________________ **Date of Visit:** ________________________
Doctor / Specialist: __________________ **Clinic / Hospital:** ____________________

Reason for Visit: _________________________

SYMPTOM SUMMARY (TO DISCUSS) *(List key concerns since last visit)*

QUESTIONS FOR THE DOCTOR

1. ____
2. ____
3. ____

DOCTOR'S OBSERVATIONS & DIAGNOSIS

MEDICATION REVIEW

Medication	Change (Start/Stop/Adjust)	Dosage	Notes

TREATMENT PLAN / RECOMMENDATIONS

☐ Physical Therapy ☐ Lifestyle Changes ☐ New Medication
☐ Tests Required ☐ Specialist Referral ☐ Other: _______

Details:

TESTS & RESULTS

Test	Date	Result	Notes

FOLLOW-UP PLAN

Next Appointment Date: ____________________

Things to Monitor Until Next Visit:

____

Pro Care Insight:
Clear communication with healthcare providers leads to better treatment decisions and improved patient outcomes.

Final 90-Day Safety Summary & Care Insights

(Complete at the End of Your Tracking Period)

TRACKING PERIOD

Start Date: ______________________________
End Date: ______________________________

OVERALL INCIDENT SUMMARY

- Total Falls: ___________
- Total Near-Falls: ___________
- Total Freezing Episodes: ___________

SAFETY TREND OVER 90 DAYS

Overall safety has:

☐ Improved
☐ Remained Stable
☐ Declined

KEY RISK PATTERNS IDENTIFIED

- Most common fall trigger:

- Most common freezing trigger:

- Most dangerous situation:

- Most frequent location of incidents:

HIGH-RISK TIMES

- Time of day with highest risk:
  ☐ Morning ☐ Afternoon ☐ Evening ☐ Night
- Specific time (if known): ______________________

FREEZING EPISODE INSIGHTS

- Frequency over time:
  ☐ Decreased ☐ Stable ☐ Increased
- Severity trend:
  ☐ Improved ☐ Same ☐ Worsened
- Most common activity during freezing:

FALL ANALYSIS

- Fall frequency over time:
  ☐ Decreased ☐ Stable ☐ Increased
- Injuries occurred: ☐ Yes ☐ No

Details: ____

MEDICATION OBSERVATIONS

- Medication taken on time:
  ☐ Always ☐ Mostly ☐ Sometimes ☐ Rarely
- Wearing-off periods:
  ☐ Reduced ☐ Stable ☐ Increased
- Link between medication and incidents:

ENVIRONMENTAL RISK SUMMARY

☐ Poor lighting
☐ Cluttered spaces
☐ Slippery surfaces
☐ Uneven flooring

Other: ____

EARLY WARNING SIGNS OBSERVED

☐ Increased freezing
☐ Reduced balance
☐ Slower movement
☐ Increased fatigue
☐ Reduced walking confidence

KEY INSIGHTS & LESSONS

What have you learned over these 90 days?

CAREGIVER REFLECTION

- Biggest challenge:

- Most helpful change made:

- What worked well:

- What needs improvement:

CAREGIVER WELL-BEING CHECK

- Average Stress Level (1–10): ________
- Average Energy Level (1–10): ________

What helped you cope the most:

ACTION PLAN GOING FORWARD

- Continue doing:
- Improve or adjust:
- Additional safety steps:

DOCTOR DISCUSSION NOTES

Use this summary during your next appointment:

A MESSAGE TO CAREGIVERS

Your dedication over these past weeks has made a real difference.
Every observation, every note, every effort—you are helping create a safer and more supportive environment.

You are not just tracking events—you are preventing them.

Share this summary with your healthcare provider for better care decisions.

Closing Message for Caregivers

Caring for someone with Parkinson's disease is a journey that requires patience, compassion, and strength. While the road may not always be easy, the care and dedication you provide make a meaningful difference in the life of the person you support.

This logbook was created to help you stay organized, recognize patterns, and communicate important information with healthcare providers. More importantly, it is a reminder that you do not have to carry every detail in your memory alone.

Each note you write represents the attention, kindness, and commitment you give every day.

Remember to care for yourself as well. Rest when you can, ask for support when needed, and recognize the incredible role you are playing.

Your effort matters. Your compassion matters. And the support you provide truly makes a difference.

Take this journey one day at a time.

A Small Request From the Author

Thank you for choosing the **Parkinson's Fall & Freezing Logbook**

Caring for someone living with Parkinson's disease is a journey that requires patience, strength, and compassion. The notes you have recorded in this journal represent the time, attention, and care you give each day.

I sincerely hope this logbook has helped you stay organized, track important information, and support the person you care for with greater confidence.

A Small Request

If you found this logbook helpful, I would truly appreciate it if you could take a moment to leave a short review on Amazon.

Your feedback helps other caregivers discover tools that may make their caregiving journey a little easier.

Even a brief review sharing your experience can make a meaningful difference.

Thank you again for the care and compassion you provide every day.

Daniel Harper
Author, *Caregiver Support Series*

www.ingramcontent.com/pod-product-compliance
Lightning Source LLC
LaVergne TN
LVHW082341200926
848481LV00012B/3408